EAT TO WIN®

FOR PERMANENT FAT LOSS

ALSO BY ROBERT HAAS

Eat to Win

Eat to Succeed

Forever Fit (coauthored with Cher)

Eat Smart, Think Smart

Permanent Remissions

EAT TO WIN®

FOR PERMANENT FAT LOSS

The Revolutionary Fat-Burning Diet
for Peak Mental and Physical Performance
and Optimum Health

Robert Haas, M.S.

Recipes by Kristin Massey

Harmony Books
New York

Published by Harmony Books, 201 East 50th Street, New York, New York 10022. Member of the Crown Publishing Group.

Random House, Inc. New York, Toronto, London, Sydney, Auckland

www.randomhouse.com

Harmony Books is a registered trademark and Harmony Books Colophon is a trademark of Random House, Inc.

Design: Meryl Sussman Levavi/Digitext, Inc.

Printed in the United States of America

Library of Congress Cataloging-in-Publication Data
Haas, Robert
    Eat to win for permanent fat loss : the revolutionary fat-burning diet for peak mental & physical performance and optimum health / Robert Haas.—1st ed.
        p. cm.
    1. Reducing diets.   2. Reducing diets—Recipes.   3. Functional foods.
    4. Athletes—Nutrition.   I. Title.
    RM222.2.H2125   2000
    613.2'5—dc21   99-049802

ISBN 0-609-60454-6

10 9 8 7 6 5 4 3 2 1

First Edition

To My Parents

CONTENTS

ACKNOWLEDGMENTS

I would like to thank the following people for their help in making this book a reality: Patty Gift, Chip Gibson, and Linda Lowenthal for their suggestions, comments, and recommendations during the writing of this book; Arielle Ford for helping me find Ling Lucas; Ling Lucas for recognizing the importance of this book and bringing it to Harmony; Steve Diamond for his software programming; and Kristin Massey, who brought impeccable taste to this book with her outstanding culinary skills.

INTRODUCTION

A book like this comes along only twice in a lifetime.

Back in the dark ages of sports nutrition—circa 1980—athletes and active people had no idea that specific foods, beverages, and dietary supplements could help burn off excess body fat, boost energy and endurance, sharpen reflexes, and maximize muscular development. In fact, most coaches, trainers, and team physicians believed that nutrition played only a minor role, at best, in fueling the fires of stamina, endurance, and peak athletic performance.

Were they ever wrong!

Tennis superstars Ivan Lendl and Martina Navratilova, like many other professional athletes during the 1980s, found religion in a new dietary doctrine. Their bible: a book I'd written called *Eat to Win*. Each became a true believer, won over after following a radical sports nutrition system that helped them shed excess body fat, build muscle, and achieve boundless energy and endurance. They publicly credited the *Eat to Win* plan with helping them lose excess body fat and boost their energy levels to dominate their sport and decimate their opponents.

In 1992, after winning an Olympic gold medal in the heptathlon event, Jackee Joyner-Kersee publicly recommended the *Eat to Win* plan to all aspiring Olympic athletes. Jackee's record includes three number-one rankings in the long jump and five more in the heptathlon and also two more Olympic gold medals, a silver and two bronzes, and another four gold medals in the outdoor World championships.

U.S. Olympic skiers, professional golfers, world-heavyweight boxers, football and baseball pros, race car drivers, swimmers, soccer players, and other martial artists, Wall Street traders, television and motion picture celebrities, and recording artists joined the growing ranks of eat-to-winners. Some athletes used the *Eat to Win* plan to earn a coveted entry in the *Guinness Book of World Records*. One physically challenged athlete, who had lost a leg to cancer, embraced the *Eat to Win* plan to help him run across the country.

Athletes past their prime competitive years soon discovered the rejuvenating powers of the *Eat to Win* plan. Golf legend Jack Nicklaus and Wimbledon champion Fred Stolle used the plan to shed difficult-to-lose pounds they had gained over the years. Tennis champions Stan Smith, Gene Mayer, and Harold Solomon embraced the plan to give them more energy and thereby prolong their professional careers. Today, former world-champion boxer George Foreman publicly recommends my dietary plan to all aspiring young athletes who want to lose excess body fat and gain a competitive advantage over opponents.

Despite the unrivaled track record of the *Eat to Win* plan, members of the American Dietetic Association and the American Medical Association disputed the value of eating a special diet to boost athletic performance and endurance. Instead, they recommended that a "balanced" diet of choices made from the common food groups was the best way for all people, including athletes, to eat. Their idea of a balanced diet included plenty of animal protein—a recommendation that opened the door to the protein pushers.

The advent of the protein pushers—diet book authors who promoted high intakes of animal protein foods for weight loss and better health—proved to be a major step backward in the evolution of nutritional science. Several physicians and self-proclaimed nutritionists (who, themselves, clearly carry body fat levels that exceed federal health guidelines) wrote self-help books touting the power of high-protein diets for athletes and couch potatoes alike. Carbohydrates, they maintained, could cripple sports performance and endurance while making people fat; protein and fat, they alleged, should form the foundation of a healthy and slimming diet. The protein pushers seduced a trusting public with sweet promises of permanent fat loss they couldn't keep. Worse yet, they touted the virtues of a performance-robbing diet based on such artery-clogging foods as filet mignon, ground beef, pastrami, mayonnaise, cheese, bacon, and heavy cream.

Instead of giving people a healthy way to lose weight and gain fitness, the protein pushers may have given their readers a head start on cardiovascular disease, breast, colon and prostate cancer, and osteoporosis. A growing body of research has linked all of these serious health problems to high-protein and/or high-fat diets.

A few diet book authors have been able to see an individual tree or two, but none has succeeded in showing readers the entire weight-loss forest. *Eat to Win for Permanent Fat Loss* aims to do that. It explains for the first time exactly *how* we lose body fat, *why* we lose body fat, which foods rev up and shut down the body's fat-burning furnace. It reveals why eating foods that control the body's glycogen (stored carbohydrate) level is the key to achieving permanent fat loss and regulating appetite and satiety. You will learn exactly how and why your body uses carbohydrates, proteins, and fats the way it does, which foods add fat to your body and which ones do not. For the first time in your life, the secrets of permanent fat loss will be within your grasp.

The nutritional strategies for achieving lifetime slimness and boosting physical and mental performance are based on my research with world champion athletes and ordinary people and on the findings of thousands of research studies published during the last twenty years. *Eat to Win for Permanent Fat Loss* is the evolutionary product of the original *Eat to Win* plan. It is the fat-burning, high-energy nutrition bible for the new century.

Eat to Win for Permanent Fat Loss introduces the most advanced dietary strategy for fat burning and optimal fitness and health—*The Ultimate Ratio.* The Ultimate Ratio combines power foods from the two healthiest diets in the world: the Mediterranean and Asian diets. I call this hybrid the "Mediterrasian" diet. In addition, the Ultimate Ratio contains a new generation of scientifically advanced functional foods and beverages. If you want to transform a Model-T body into a Ferrari physique, the Ultimate Ratio can help you do it better, faster, safer, and more efficiently than any other eating strategy.

The Ultimate Ratio combines the following four categories to create a single super diet:

1. *Traditional Foods.* The Ultimate Ratio emphasizes the traditional foods eaten by Mediterranean and Asian people—including fish, shellfish, legumes, garlic, onions, olive oil, soy foods, vegetables, pasta, fresh fruits, and chocolate.

2. *Traditional Beverages.* When first I analyzed the everyday beverages of the Mediterranean and Asian diets, I discovered that they are richly endowed with thousands of compounds called *phytonutrients*. Phytonutrients impart color, flavor, and aroma to vegetables, fruits, and herbs. They make red grapes red, blueberries blue, and green beans green. The give garlic and onions their characteristic aroma. Once in the body, they can help prevent and mitigate the degenerative diseases that afflict many people, including cancer, heart disease, diabetes, and osteoporosis. Among the most common beverages were cocoa and chocolate, coffee, green and black teas, fermented rice (sake), and fermented grapes (wine). Many of the phytonutrients present in cocoa beans, tea leaves, and coffee beans provide powerful antioxidants that can prevent and relieve muscle soreness, boost energy and athletic performance, protect joints from inflammation, and reduce the risk of infection and illness.

3. *Functional Foods.* Modern food science has moved beyond traditional foods, with the creation of functional foods and beverages. Food scientists have produced a number of functional foods that contain concentrated protein and phytonutrients derived from the soybean. There are dozens of these meat-replacement products sold in ordinary supermarkets and natural foods markets that will help you and your family eat according to the Ultimate Ratio without giving up the taste of the foods you already love. This new generation of soy foods is as delicious to children as it is to adults.

4. *Functional Beverages.* These drinks, chock full of compounds now being tested by the National Cancer Institute's Diet and Cancer branch, contain a number of natural compounds that will help you burn body fat, boost mental and physical performance, and reduce the risk of getting such serious diseases as cancer, atherosclerosis, and adult-onset diabetes. I started making functional beverages from raw nutrients in my own kitchen nearly twenty years ago. Thanks to current food technology, you don't have to make such beverages from scratch because you can now buy them in natural foods stores and vitamin shops.

Our children are the athletic champions of tomorrow, and because every child needs peak performance nutrition to do better in all areas of life, I've designed the Ultimate Ratio for the whole family. Children past the age of twelve on up to adults and senior citizens will now be able to enjoy greater energy, increased physical and mental stamina, and permanent fat loss thanks to the fifteen years of new research and discoveries I've incorporated in this book. Whether you eat in or dine out, you and your family will be able to enjoy a new breakthrough in achieving permanent fat loss and improved physical performance with the Ultimate Ratio.

My research into fat loss and peak performance nutrition began in college, shortly after Uncle Sam invited me to join his Army. At my physical exam, a military physician stared intently at the blood pressure gauge on the band wrapped snugly around my left arm. I saw his forehead jerk upward. "Is there a problem?" I asked. "You bet your life there is!" he replied. "Your blood pressure is dangerously high. You are a prime candidate for a stroke, young man!" The U.S. Army classified me as unfit for military service.

That was the first time I learned I had a serious health problem. Subsequently I also learned that the drugs my doctor prescribed to treat my high blood pressure carried devastating side effects that could be debilitating and even as life-threatening as the condition they were prescribed to treat. My physician told me there was no cure for my high blood pressure and that I would have to stay on medication for the rest of my life—a life that suddenly seemed very precarious.

I felt I could do something about my condition, and believed that diet played a role in causing it—despite the fact that my physician told me my diet had nothing to do with my high blood pressure. So I began to research the relationship between diet, health, fitness, and disease. Up to that point, I had followed the diet my coaches prescribed: lots of protein—the same type of diet that today's protein-pushing diet-book authors promote! As I discovered, it was precisely the kind of diet that got me into trouble. What I discovered about nutrition not only reversed my health and weight problem but also became part of a diet revolution, changing the way millions of people ate the world over, including the world's best athletes.

What practical benefits have I reaped from my nutritional research?

- I look fifteen years younger than my age.
- I rarely get sick.
- I'm rarely tired.
- My total cholesterol level is 140 mg/100 milliliters (ml) of blood. My HDL cholesterol is 65 mg/100 ml of blood.
- I have a much lower percentage of body fat and a higher percentage of muscle tissue than I did at age eighteen. My BMI (*body-mass index*— a measure of body fatness) is 21. (See page 29 for the way to calculate the BMI.)

- I enjoy an extraordinary level of fitness, far above that which most middle-age males possess.
- I can work long hours at a stretch—often putting in ten to fourteen hours a day in research and writing in addition to daily exercise. My mental focus and concentration remain laser-sharp.

Eat to Win for Permanent Fat Loss is the culmination of my studies and years of clinical research to help you achieve permanent fat loss, optimal fitness, and better health.

Do you or your children aspire to a career in professional sports? Eating according to the Ultimate Ratio will greatly increase the chances of attaining that goal. World-class athletes require world-class sports nutrition counseling—a strategy often missing from the elite athlete's training plan. Athletes may benefit from the advice of a coach, strength trainer, sports psychologist, and physiotherapist, but they rarely receive the kind of sports nutrition counseling that can unify and enhance these other training disciplines. This deficiency robs professional athletes of their ultimate performance potential. In addition, elite junior athletes rarely experience the developmental advantages that cutting-edge sports nutrition can afford them. Many talented juniors frequently fail to live up to their promise because they could not sustain the requisite peak mental and physical performance required to advance to the next level.

Through my experience and research, I have been able to pinpoint the nutritional elements that hold back athletic achievement. Having worked extensively with elite athletes often as insecure as they are gifted, I have discovered how to motivate them and coax significant gains from them. Although I can't work personally with you, I can do the next best thing: give you and your family the dietary blueprint for success in all areas of your active life.

As I watch professional athletes compete today, I am often perplexed at the unscientific way most of them still eat, and the excess body fat that many carry around to their detriment. Whenever I counsel junior athletes, I am struck by the lack of sound nutritional guidance offered by their coaches and parents. These are America's future champions, yet they are eating to *lose*.

Are their role models any different? In my opinion, a number of tennis, golf, football, and baseball superstars sport unacceptably high levels of body fat for elite athletes. Lack of fitness—as evidenced by repeated muscle cramps, muscle pulls, and bouts of heat exhaustion—have hurt the careers of these otherwise gifted competitors.

As these athletes and those who will one day take their places strive to be the best they can, they will increasingly need to push the limits of human performance and endurance to new levels. The Ultimate Ratio can help them achieve these goals. As champions, they should aspire to nothing less.

It's time for you and your family to reap the benefits of this revolutionary eating plan. You're about to experience the exhilarating thrill of peak physical and mental performance while you redesign your body from the inside out.

It's time for you to learn how to eat to win—for *permanent* fat loss.

Visit the Eat to Win web site at: www.e2win.com.

THE REVOLUTIONARY
FAT-BURNING DIET

1

EAT YOUR WAY TO THE TOP

WITH THE ULTIMATE RATIO

A re you looking to make a meal out of the competition?

What's important to you—speed? size? strength? What about energy, endurance, mental focus, and vitality? Or, maybe it's losing body fat and looking great.

I am going to show you how to accomplish all of these goals with a revolutionary eating plan that I have used to help world-class and recreational athletes of all ages slim down, shape up, and succeed in their chosen sport or physical activity. Make no mistake: All of us—even couch potatoes—need to eat as if we were athletes in order to burn fat and tone muscle.

Although most of us will never win a Wimbledon championship or an Olympic gold medal, we can all aspire to physical and mental excellence. No matter if you are eight or eighty, I will show you how to achieve these goals on the court, at the office, and in the classroom. You'll even learn to love your bathroom scale. From this moment on, you will never again just eat to eat— you will eat to *win*.

THE ULTIMATE RATIO

Why do the people I advise consistently beat the odds and conquer the competition—while others with similar levels of training and skill turn in second-rate performances? Why do my clients lose significant amounts of body fat and keep it off, while other people lose and regain it in a vicious, repetitive cycle?

The answer is simple: I've helped my clients eat their way to the top of their chosen sport or profession with a performance-enhancing nutrition system I call the Ultimate Ratio. The Ultimate Ratio accomplishes far more than any other diet or performance-based eating plan can because it:

1. *Leads to permanent fat loss* by forcing the body to burn excess fat, while it also maximizes energy, vitality, and strength;
2. *Transforms muscle cells* into potent powerhouses that will make you go faster, higher, and farther;
3. *Supercharges the mind-body connection*—a powerful bond that links physical and mental fitness to enhance sports performance, reaction time, alertness, mental focus, and problem solving.

The Ultimate Ratio has been tested in recreational and world champion athletes; it has helped all of them achieve new heights of performance and endurance. It offers a better chance for permanent fat loss than any other eating plan because it satisfies people's taste for fat while also helping the body burn excess fat.

The Ultimate Ratio can help ordinary people improve their personal performance as much or more than it can help the world's most gifted athletes. While it can shave tenths of a second off an Olympic athlete's time in the 400-meter dash—often the difference between winning the gold or silver medal—it can shave *minutes* off your personal best in a 10k road race. Or it can simply help you make it through the day with more energy.

The Ultimate Ratio will help you work out longer and harder at your health club, play tougher tennis, or shoot better golf. It will help you think faster, enjoy greater mental energy, and improve concentration. For kids and teens, eating according to the Ultimate Ratio can mean making the soccer, basketball, tennis, or football team, getting better grades and higher test scores in school, and preventing weight gain and obesity. Eating according to the Ultimate Ratio will help maximize your child's full potential for growth, health, and fitness.

Just ten years ago, eating according to the Ultimate Ratio was time-consuming and more difficult than it is today. Thanks to the development of a new category of functional foods, getting the right nutrients in the right amounts is now simpler, faster, and more satisfying in taste.

EATING TO WIN MAKES MIRACLES HAPPEN

There are people who believe that great tennis champions like Ivan Lendl, Martina Navratilova, and Andre Agassi are born, not made. It is true that most athletic champions are genetically gifted in various ways. But the skill levels of most elite athletes at or near the top of each sport are comparable. A matter of a few hundredths of a second in a foot race or a few key points in a tennis match often determine the difference between being the champion or the runner-up. And that's where eating to win can make *the* difference. Skill and genetic endowment, important as they may be, are often not enough on any given day to overcome a determined and equally endowed opponent. The top pros know this and constantly search for a way to gain a competitive advantage. Nutritional science gives them such an advantage, and it can do the same for you in all areas of your life.

In Ivan Lendl's case, hard work, perseverance, and a demanding training schedule gave him the endurance, confidence, and ability to dominate men's professional tennis longer than any player in history (a remarkable 270 weeks at number one). In 1983, Lendl's dream of dominating men's professional tennis remained unrealized and he considered quitting the sport. His manager, Jerry Solomon, called me in a state of distress to ask if I could help Ivan achieve his world-champion potential, as I had done with Martina Navratilova. I told him I believed I could, and shortly after I began working with Ivan he rose to number one in the world and stayed at the top for over five straight years—following the same outstanding pattern of success that Martina had enjoyed with cutting-edge sports nutrition—*my way.*

Andre Agassi needed to jump-start his career after a four-year decline. No one questioned his natural talent or powerful technique, but sports pundits had totally written off Andre, who was losing consistently to opponents he should have beaten. So Andre began training harder, eating wiser, and using a number of peak performance nutrients, which I will tell you about in chapter 6. This strategy boosted Andre's reflexes and mind-body connection to new heights while helping him melt off excess body fat and preserve his muscle mass during fat loss. The result? Andre revived a stalled career at the "late" age of 29 and regained the number-one ranking in the world. As John McEnroe observed, "This proves that miracles really do happen in sports."

GLYCOGEN:
THE KEY TO PERMANENT FAT LOSS

When you enjoy the carbohydrate-rich foods of the Ultimate Ratio, you can eat them to your heart's content without fear of getting fat. Why? Because of *glycogen*—the body's storage form of carbohydrate and the key to permanent fat loss.

Here's what nearly all diet book authors fail to understand about permanent fat loss: When you learn how to regulate your body's glycogen levels, you will control how much fat you will burn each day, every day. The Ultimate Ratio puts you in complete control of your own fat burning—permanently. How does this remarkable slimming process work?

Under normal conditions, your body will *not* convert the carbohydrates you eat to fat (it also resists converting pure protein and alcohol to fat as well). Instead, your body, in its wisdom, increases its burning of carbohydrates proportionally—the more of them you eat, the more your body burns them for fuel or stores the excess in the liver and muscles as glycogen. That's why eating the Ultimate Ratio recommended carbohydrates will not add fat to your body. Eating too many carbohydrates may stop you from burning off the body fat you have already stored around your thighs, butt, and stomach, but eating recommended Ultimate Ratio carbohydrates will not add fat to your body. Only dietary fat can do that.

Most diet book authors do not understand this concept, and so they devise unhealthy high-fat/high-protein diets designed to deprive the body of its glycogen in a misguided attempt to "fool" the body into burning fat. In the short run, high-fat diets dehydrate the body, leading to a false sense of fat loss. Eventually, these diets fail when carbohydrate cravings inevitably return. Why? It's because the body and brain demand carbohydrates for peak performance. Over the long run, your body craves carbohydrates because they are the optimal source of energy and satiety.

Carbohydrate usage, whether burned for fuel or stored as glycogen, is so closely controlled by the body that even if you overeat carbohydrates on occasion, you will not become obese. Your body will simply increase carbohydrate oxidation (burning for fuel) or store the excess in your glycogen tank. In fact, you can eat 2,000 to 3,000 carbohydrate calories each day before your body will even begin to convert the excess calories to fat. The Ultimate Ratio shows you which foods will help control your body's glycogen levels to lead you directly to a lifetime of slenderness.

THE ULTIMATE RATIO DELIVERS PERMANENT WEIGHT LOSS

Dietitians, psychologists, most commercial weight-loss organizations, and other health-care providers all agree on at least one thing: to lose weight, you should count calories and eat less. While this sounds logical and looks good on paper, it simply doesn't work for most people. Dieting by counting calories and restricting food intake is self-destructive. Just as it's impossible to hold your breath forever, you simply cannot maintain the discipline to restrict calories for a lifetime. So it is nearly impossible to sustain weight loss permanently by following this antiquated advice.

Our taste for fat—which is the *only* nutrient the body stores directly and immediately as body fat—is nearly as powerful as our drive for food itself. Long before civilization as we know it existed, this drive kept our ancestors from starving during periods of famine. Today, it keeps us from achieving optimal health and reaching our perfect weight. It all comes down to this: Mother Nature has given you a taste for fat so strong that it conflicts with your desire to be thin. Trying to adopt what is essentially an unnatural behavior (food deprivation) will lead to failure most of the time. And those are odds that no one should have to face. With the Ultimate Ratio, you can finally beat the odds.

When you simply cut calories and eliminate tasty foods from your diet, you set your conscious mind and innate drive for satiety at odds with each other. This creates a self-defeating conflict, which virtually all diet experts ignore despite a wealth of clinical evidence corroborating the fact that *most people will not deny themselves the tastes they love, even at the risk of succumbing to such health problems as obesity, cardiovascular disease, cancer, hypertension, and adult-onset diabetes.* Published scientific evidence clearly demonstrates that a majority of us lack the willpower to override our preference for the taste of fat.

Okay, so calorie counting and food deprivation don't work. What about such extremes as high-protein diets and low-fat diets—will those lead to permanent fat loss? After you've read chapter 2, you will understand how high-protein diets must inevitably fail because they contain too much fat and they deprive your body of sufficient carbohydrates to keep binge eating at bay. You will learn that very low-fat (10 percent) diets don't lead most people to permanent weight loss because they conflict with your inborn preference for the taste of fat. You will also discover why simply cutting calories without changing the composition of your diet leads to a vicious cycle of gaining and losing weight. Most important, you will learn how the Ultimate Ratio can help you reach your perfect weight by allowing you to enjoy the taste of fat. It is now possible to enjoy many of your favorite "fattening" foods—even fast foods—thanks to a new class of very healthy and slimming food products called functional foods.

Once you have lost all of your excess body fat with the Ultimate Ratio, you will literally look and feel like a new person. And with your newly redesigned body comes the power to resist the temptation to cheat. Only then will you really understand what I have been telling my clients for years:

NOTHING TASTES AS GOOD AS THIN FEELS!

FUNCTIONAL FOODS

ON THE CUTTING EDGE OF SPORTS, NUTRITION, AND PERMANENT FAT LOSS

When is a food not just a food? When it's a *functional* food.

Swiss pharmacist Henri Nestlé concocted one of the world's first functional foods in 1867. He paved the way for bottle feeding by inventing baby formula. Nestlé's babyfood-in-a-bottle idea gave millions of infants who would have died without their mother's milk a second chance at life.

Modern functional foods, as dietary supplement manufacturers like to call these new health and fitness enhancers (drug companies prefer the term "nutraceuticals"), represent an exploding market conservatively estimated at more than $29 billion a year in the United States.

Most of us have been eating rudimentary types of functional foods for years in the form of vitamin-fortified breakfast cereals, iron-enriched breads; and vitamin A- and D-fortified milk. Such fortification was done to prevent nutritional deficiencies. Permanent fat loss and boosting athletic and mental fitness never crossed the mind of these food-fortifying manufacturers.

A NEW FOOD GROUP FOR A NEW CENTURY

I know that to many people, soy is a four-letter word. It's not surprising. Their parents didn't serve them soy "hot dogs," "hamburgers," and "milkshakes," and so most of them don't buy them or serve them to their families. And that's a shame—because you can burn fat and build a better body with soy.

Thanks to such food manufacturers as Morningstar Farms, Yves Veggie Cuisine, Boca Burger, and Worthington Foods (see appendix III, page 225), you can bring home a grocery bag full of fast food treats that will make your family happy and their bodies healthy. For the first time in history, you and your family can enjoy eating "meat"—quite literally to your heart's content—while burning body fat and preventing such diet-related diseases as certain types of cancer and atherosclerosis, which gain a foothold in the body during childhood.

Soy food products and the new soy shake mixes (called soy "cocktails" or soy "beverages"), which contain powerful phytonutrients and antioxidants, have recently gained the respect of leading health organizations such as the National Cancer Institute and the approval of consumers. Beef lovers may call soy "mystery meat," but I call it a peak performance miracle. The athletic champions of the twenty-first century will eat to win with soy protein.

Some soy products fare better than others when it comes to providing high amounts of disease-fighting compounds called *isoflavones.* Unfortunately, a great deal of the isoflavone content of soy is washed out during commercial preparation of some soy meat substitutes. Several brands of veggie burgers and vegetarian chili mixes use soy protein made by alcohol extraction, a process that diminishes soy's disease-fighting isoflavone content. If you stick with the soy products recommended in this book, you will avoid using isoflavone-depleted products.

By now you are probably quite curious about these amazing foods and beverages. Look at pages 186 and 167 for two of my favorite functional food (soy-based) recipes: the Big Max Burger and the Purple Cow shake. Here is a McDonald's Big Mac–like burger that can help prevent cancer, heart disease, and obesity while boosting fitness and building strong bones and muscles. And for kids who don't like broccoli or the color green, introduce them to purple—the Purple Cow.

THE POWER OF FUNCTIONAL FOODS AND DRINKS

The *Big Max Burger* and the *Purple Cow* are just two examples of my favorite functional foods and drinks that have helped many of my clients reach their ideal weights. Teens and adults alike enjoy the delicious flavors of these healthy fast-food recipes while obtaining their nutritional benefits, such as lowered blood cholesterol and denser bones. These recipes supply the phytonutrients, antioxidants, vitamins, and minerals that can help atone for the nutritional sins of those who don't or won't eat their spinach.

Many people have never heard of functional foods and drinks, and the mere mention that these foods contain chemicals—*phyto*chemicals (the naturally occurring disease-fighting compounds found in fruits and vegetables)—is enough to cause the uninformed consumer to avoid them. People forget that every known substance has a chemical formula; it's the natural chemicals in foods that fuel the chemical processing plants in our bodies. Functional foods contain a rich supply of peak-performance phytochemicals and can help balance the less-than-perfect diets most people eat.

Several years ago, the National Cancer Institute started a special branch that studies phytochemicals and functional foods. Coffee retail giant Starbucks recently jumped into the functional-food fray by offering java with a jolt of extra protein, vitamins, and minerals. Coffee itself is a healthful drink (unless you are sensitive to caffeine) that contains natural anticancer phytonutrients. In my opinion, functional foods and beverages are the future of peak-performance nutrition. Fortunately, the future is already here.

One important caveat concerning functional foods: Peak-performance nutrition relies on the interplay of many compounds in foods; scientists cannot yet re-create that complexity in a capsule or drink. Functional foods cannot supplant the nutritional completeness of whole, natural foods. On the other hand, a single functional food or drink can help boost energy and mental focus while it promotes fat loss and protects against such serious health problems as cancer, heart disease, adult-onset diabetes, and osteoporosis.

The 1980s and 1990s were the decades of avoiding foods to avoid disease. I hope the twenty-first century will be a time of embracing Ultimate Ratio traditional and functional foods to achieve permanent fat loss, peak performance, and optimum health.

THE ULTIMATE RATIO'S "MEDITERRASIAN" ADVANTAGE

The Ultimate Ratio incorporates the most powerful nutritional components of the two healthiest diets in the world—the Mediterranean and Asian diets.

No other way of eating can give you the health and fat-loss benefits of this "Mediterrasian" eating plan.

The Ultimate Ratio provides your body with the ultimate biochemistry for peak mental and physical performance. Moreover, the Ultimate Ratio contains the ideal mixture of protein, fat, and carbohydrate, building muscle and strengthening the immune system.

The Ultimate Ratio contains an exceptionally high concentration of phytonutrients—found only in vegetables, fruits, and herbs. Phytonutrients are the most powerful disease-preventing nutrients known—many are more powerful than the most potent vitamins. Phytonutrients, including *lycopene* (found in tomatoes, watermelon, lobster), *genistein* (found in soy foods and beverages), and phenolics (found in most fruits and vegetables) can reduce muscle damage from strenuous exercise and protect against cancer and other serious health problems.

THE ULTIMATE RATIO'S MIND-BODY CONNECTION

Have you ever heard the expression "Be the ball?" That is Zen-speak used by sports psychologists for becoming one with your surroundings—a state of mind-body unity you can achieve with proper training and the Ultimate Ratio. It is a state of "oneness" that all sports champions understand because they've been there from time to time. When home-run hitters or tennis champions no longer see the bat or tennis racquet as being separate from their arms, when they visualize the oncoming ball as part of the process of play rather than a separate entity, they have achieved mind-body unity. They are one with the ball, the bat, or the racquet at that moment. They are not thinking. They are feeling. They are being.

When athletes describe their mental state during peak performance, chances are they'll refer to it as a type of mind-body connection. Most have no idea how or why they made this unified connection. And, unfortunately, they can't re-create it on demand.

There are only two ways athletes can achieve this mind-body connection. The first is through years of repetitive practice of an activity or movement until they have perfected it and it becomes "second nature" to them. The second, more immediate way, is by eating a diet that boosts the brain's supply of "smart nutrients," facilitating communication between the brain, nerves, and muscles—the same ones Ivan Lendl used to dominate men's professional tennis for five straight years.

The neuromuscular science behind the mind-body connection is well established. Quite simply, food contains the basic building blocks that the body uses to manufacture chemical messengers (called neurotransmitters) that help the brain and muscles communicate with each other. When you eat according to the Ultimate Ratio, you supply your brain and muscles with the food and nutrients in the proper proportions they need to strengthen and improve the mind-body connection. With sports training, that connection—commonly called muscle memory—is continually reinforced and grows stronger each day. Facilitating muscle memory will help improve your golf swing, tennis backhand, and your ability to assimilate and execute coaching and training techniques aimed at making you a better athlete and competitor. Recent published research has shown that the nutritional compounds in the Ultimate Ratio can significantly improve your tennis strokes and golf swing.

Achieving a dynamic mind-body connection is the surest and fastest way to realize the maximum mental and physical potential dictated by your own genetics. If you want to consistently tap into your full mind-body potential, you should enjoy the smart foods and nutrients of the Ultimate Ratio.

MAXIMIZING MUSCULAR PERFORMANCE

Like tiny high-performance car engines, every muscle cell in your body requires the ideal fuel mixture, fuel additives, and coolant to run at optimum performance levels. In order to keep up with energy demands, each cell must have a steady supply of the right stuff in the right proportion or ratio. Too much or too little protein or the wrong type of fat or carbohydrate can throw a monkey wrench into the cellular machinery responsible for peak athletic performance. Few professional athletes and even fewer ordinary people regularly reap the rewards of having all three elements—the perfect fuel mixture, the right fuel additives, proper lubricants—in the right place at the right time. Why not?

Because no one has told them how to do it until now.

When you eat according to the Ultimate Ratio, you begin to efficiently tune the millions of cellular engines in your muscles, transforming them from Volkswagens into Ferraris. When you "feed your machine" with the

Ultimate Ratio you will achieve the Holy Grail of athletic training—the performance edge.

REDESIGNING YOUR BODY—FROM THE INSIDE OUT

The Ultimate Ratio works quickly and effectively because it literally redesigns your body from the inside out. Your muscles will become more biochemically fit to burn off excess fat and carry you faster, higher, and farther in your chosen sport or exercise. The results will show—inside and out:

Inside: Your blood is the mirror of your body. That's why I recommend that everyone have a simple and inexpensive blood chemistry profile test (see page 215) when they begin the Ultimate Ratio. After just one month, a follow-up test will reveal some very favorable changes in your cholesterol, triglycerides (blood fats), and glucose levels. These values can reveal many things about the state of your health and your biologic age. For example, healthy children generally have cholesterol values between 120 and 140 and fasting blood glucose and triglyceride values under 80 (all values are typically reported in milligrams per 100 milliliters of blood). Within four to eight weeks after you begin the Ultimate Ratio, you will notice that your blood chemistry numbers begin to approach those of a child's. In essence, you have begun the process of deaging your blood. That translates into better health and improved fitness potential.

Outside: Shortly after you begin the Ultimate Ratio, you will acquire the energy, stamina, and endurance to play and train harder and faster. Your skin will begin to look healthier and more youthful; your excess body fat will melt away to reveal newly toned muscle. Your freshly sculpted body will show the unmistakable hallmarks of someone who eats according to the Ultimate Ratio.

BOOSTING YOUR THREE MOST IMPORTANT ENERGY SOURCES

In theory, the Ultimate Ratio could boost muscular strength, power, and speed far beyond the level enjoyed by today's Olympic athletes. In reality, the body does not run at 100 percent efficiency, and so humans cannot use all of the available force out of their muscles. Doing so could break a bone or tear a tendon.

The practical limits of human performance—strength, speed, and endurance—are largely determined at the cellular level. It's really a question of how much energy, in the form of the three most important energy sources listed below, that your muscles can store and how quickly you can replenish them:

1. *ATP* (adenosine triphosphate): the universal energy molecule in all living things)
2. *Glycogen:* stored carbohydrate
3. *Triglycerides:* stored fat

Genetics plays an important role in determining the limits of your own personal performance—how much blood your heart can pump during physical activity, for example—but the foods and nutrients of the Ultimate Ratio can improve your muscles' storage and utilization of these three most important energy sources.

TAKING YOUR NEW BODY TO THE LIMIT

Success, like beauty, is in the eye of the beholder. A weekend athlete may define success as simply *finishing* a 10-kilometer race, a 26-mile marathon, or perhaps beating a weekend tennis or golf opponent for the first time in years. A world-class athlete may define success as winning an Olympic gold medal or breaking a world record. The Ultimate Ratio can help active people to reach their ideal weight and fitness goals.

2

PROTEIN INSANITY

DEBUNKING THE PROTEIN PUSHERS

R emember the 1980s—when health-conscious Americans clogged jogging paths and exercise trials instead of their arteries? How could the '80s health and fitness movement, which seemed to be enjoying such muscular growth, have atrophied so miserably? Whatever happened to those days when adults and adolescents, on average, were ten pounds lighter and restaurants served more calorically conservative portions? How on earth did we become one of the world's fattest nations?

A glut of diet doctors and health faddists has offered a tired but perennially seductive answer: Americans grew fatter because they ate too many carbohydrates and not enough protein and fat. "Most Americans are protein deficient," claims a well-known and overweight diet doctor. Another chubby high priest of high protein, who apparently lives in a nutritional twilight zone, recommends that we consume at least 30 percent of our daily calories as protein and avoid many healthful fruits and vegetables. This author offers up my favorite faux pearl of nutritional wisdom: "Fat does not make you fat." More misleading and inaccurate statements can be found in another popular high-protein diet book written by two physicians: "The actual amount of carbohydrate *required* by humans for health is *zero*"; "Most vegetable sources of protein—beans and grains—are incomplete."

Say hello to the protein pushers.

WATCH OUT FOR THE BULL

Protein pushing dates back to ancient Greece and Rome, when athletes believed that to be as strong as a bull you had to—eat bull. We can smile at such nutritional alchemy as primitive and unscientific—or can we?

Apparently, many Americans regain their appetite for bull (and the gullibility to swallow it) every decade or so. Since the early 1950s and with predictable regularity, someone has written a popular protein-pushing, carbohydrate-bashing diet book. The first generation of these books told us that carbohydrates, not calories, made us fat. A second generation of physician-authored books—"quick" weight-loss diets, "medical" diets, and diet "revolutions"—perpetuated carbo-phobia throughout the 1960s, '70s, and '80s. The American waistline continued to grow in proportion to the number of protein-pushing weight-loss books.

The current crop of high-protein diet books is really a case of old wine in new bottles. With minor variations, all of these books serve up the same tired message that recalls the dietary dogma of the 1950s, when the centerpiece of restaurant diet plates was a ground beef patty—hold the bun: Eating carbohydrates makes you chubby; eating animal protein and fat slims you down. Evidently, ancient Greek and Roman athletes were not the only ones who were full of bull.

Wouldn't it be wonderful if you could, as many of today's protein pushers promise, eat bacon, filet mignon, spareribs, ham, eggs, lamb, cheese, butter, and heavy cream to permanently lose weight and get healthier? What dieter wouldn't be seduced with the promise of enjoying such sumptuous foods at every meal? But what if the real promise of these diets was actually a multitude of diseases.

Ironically, many of today's protein pushers claim that, by eating more fat and protein and less carbohydrate, your risk of developing disease decreases. Where is the proof that their "eat-the-burger-hold-the-bun" theory works? That's one minor detail all of them have overlooked. There is none. On the other hand, a large body of published scientific studies has consistently documented the health hazards of consuming high-protein/high-fat diets.

GETTING UNHEALTHIER—ONE BITE AT A TIME

What is a high-protein diet? How does it differ from the diets consumed by ordinary Americans?

One popular high-protein diet recommends that you consume 30 percent fat, 40 percent carbohydrate, and 30 percent protein. With the exception of a more generous dose of protein, this is already quite close to the customary American diet. And most Americans are already overweight or obese. So what's the truth? Can a high-protein diet help you achieve permanent fat loss?

Not likely. High-protein diets represent a triple threat to your waistline because:

1. They promote eating calorically dense animal-protein foods such as lamb, duck, and beef, and such high-fat foods as vegetable oils, cheese, butter, cream, and food products that contain them. As you will discover, it is precisely these foods—not carbohydrates—that make you fat.

2. These foods score lower than many Ultimate Ratio complex carbohydrate foods on the satiety index, a measure of how well a food fills you up. You tend to eat these foods quickly, which usually encourages greater food and calorie consumption.

3. People tend to clean their plates on high-protein diets, no matter how much food is on the plate; this makes restaurant dining—where one is likely to be served Godzilla-sized portions—a nutritional risk and a caloric disaster.

What is the chance of permanently keeping off the weight you lose on a high-protein diet? Very small. After a brief honeymoon period during which a high-protein/high-fat diet kills your appetite and dehydrates your muscles (which gives trusting dieters a false sense of fat loss), carbohydrate cravings inevitably return—Mother Nature's way of telling your body to stop the high-protein insanity.

GET OUT OF THE HIGH-PROTEIN TWILIGHT ZONE

The protein pushers make one scientifically valid observation when they write about the health risks associated with overconsumption of sugar.

Beyond that, there is precious little information in these books that will lead you to permanent fat loss or optimal health. Although these well-meaning authors genuinely want to help solve the problem of obesity, their zeal to do so evidently interferes with their ability to thoroughly evaluate and accurately apply even the most rudimentary nutritional knowledge.

There is no published scientific proof that eating a high-protein/high-fat diet will lower the incidence of heart disease, cancer, osteoporosis, or adult-onset diabetes. None of the protein pushers can point to long-term studies of thousands of people that show a high-protein/high-fat diet leading to permanent weight loss. In fact, there are a number of published biomedical studies that suggest eating a high-protein diet can make you fat. One study, in which researchers fed lab rats a low- (5 percent) and high- (25 percent) protein diet, showed that the high-protein diet made rats 50 percent fatter than rats fed a low-protein diet of the same caloric content.

Okay, so high-protein diets make fat rats. But what about people? Published studies on free-living human populations around the world provide irrefutable evidence that people who eat diets high in animal protein and fat suffer higher rates of obesity and diet-related diseases than populations that eat less animal protein and more protein from soy and other legumes, seafood, and vegetables.

Will a high-protein/high-fat diet ultimately make *you* fatter or leaner? By the time you finish reading this chapter, you will be able to answer that question for yourself.

THE ULTIMATE RATIO IS SUPPORTED BY SCIENCE

A multitude of published scientific studies has consistently shown that diets high in phytonutrient-rich foods—the primary foods of the Ultimate Ratio plan—prevent people from becoming obese. There is abundant published evidence that diets similar to the Ultimate Ratio confer protection against heart disease, cancer, adult-onset diabetes, osteoporosis, and obesity. In fact, it is overwhelming. You will find the published proof for the scientific rationale behind the Ultimate Ratio listed in the bibliography, pages 229–256.

The news about protein is not all bad. Protein is an essential nutrient that plays a vital role in health and fitness. Learning which type of protein is best and how much you need marks the first step in learning how to eat to win with the Ultimate Ratio.

PROTEIN

FIRST, THE GOOD NEWS

Protein, when consumed in correct amounts, is a good thing. Our bodies cannot function properly without a sufficient supply of protein each day. We need a daily dose of protein because:

- Muscle tissue contains a number of proteins without which you couldn't move, run, jump, or even blink your eyes.
- Hemoglobin, the oxygen-carrying molecule that helps you run longer and farther, is made of protein.
- The enzymes that help build muscle, create energy, and burn body fat are made from protein.
- Your hair, nails, and outer layers of skin are made of protein.
- Your bones are made of protein.
- Your brain and nervous system use protein to make chemical messengers that control thought, memory, and problem solving as well as communicate with all the other organs in the body.

Thus protein itself is hardly a nutritional villain. Eating the right amount and type of protein will help you stay healthy and fit. People living in the United States and other technologically advanced countries rarely underconsume protein. If anything, they suffer from protein *surplus.* Our national love affair with high-protein foods promotes serious health problems and robs us of our true performance potential.

THEN THE BAD NEWS

Protein is a powerful and important nutrient, but it has a biochemical dark side. Protein's Jekyll and Hyde nature makes it imperative that you understand the consequences of eating the type of high-protein diet promoted by the protein pushers. If you follow their advice, eating that much protein can throw a molecular monkey wrench into your muscles, liver, and kidneys. Here's why:

Protein makes a dirty body fuel. Unlike carbohydrates and fats, protein contains nitrogen. And therein lies the problem. Instead of producing "clean" metabolic byproducts such as carbon dioxide and water (as only carbohydrates do), protein produces the nitrogenous waste products, ammonia and urea (two ammonia molecules bonded to a carbon atom). These compounds can adversely affect your immune system, rob your bones of calcium, and tax your liver and kidneys.

Protein makes an inefficient body fuel. Protein has more important jobs to do in your body than supply energy. When you need to go the extra mile—whether it's keeping up with your kids at a shopping mall or finishing a 10k race, protein provides scant energy compared to carbohydrate and fat. The reason is that your body has to expend more energy to convert protein into energy than it does for carbohydrates and fats. High-protein diets defeat peak physical performance in two ways:

   1. By drastically reducing an athlete's carbohydrate intake, they actually *increase* the daily requirement for protein. The reason is a little appreciated biochemical fact: *Carbohydrates spare protein.* During exercise and long periods of exertion your body craves carbohydrates—not protein—and it will do whatever it takes to get them, including cannibalizing your own muscle tissue. Protein from muscles can be converted to glucose, but it is an inefficient and dirty process.
   2. They literally cramp an athlete's style, because a reduced carbohydrate intake drains the body's supply of glycogen (a reserve of carbohydrate stored in the muscles and liver), thereby limiting the amount of time an athlete's muscles can perform to exhaustion.

High-Protein Diets and Urea Toxicity

Urea is the final waste product of protein metabolism. Chemical companies must use very high heat and pressure to manufacture urea, but your body can easily make urea out of ammonia and a few enzymes. In order to neutralize ammonia and urea, the body draws calcium and other minerals from bones along with water from muscle cells. The more protein you eat, the more ammonia and urea you make. High-protein diets thin your bones, predisposing you to osteoporosis later in life; they also dehydrate your body, crippling athletic performance and endurance.

Comparing the Diets: Which One Would You Pick?

HIGH-PROTEIN DIET
GLYCOGEN
0.6 g/100g

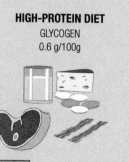

MAXIMUM WORK TIME: 60 MINUTES

MIXED DIET
GLYCOGEN
1.8 g/100g

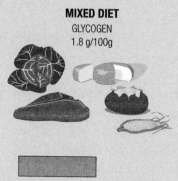

MAXIMUM WORK TIME: 120 MINUTES

ULTIMATE RATIO DIET
GLYCOGEN
3.5 g/100g

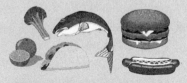

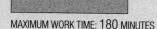

MAXIMUM WORK TIME: 180 MINUTES

The Ultimate Ratio contains all the delicious foods that most people have become accustomed to eating, including such fast foods as hamburgers, hot dogs, and tacos. The difference is that on the Ultimate Ratio plan these fast-food favorites help you burn excess body fat, build muscle, and boost mental performance. Why? Because they are made from a new generation of lower-calorie and lower-fat soy-protein foods and functional foods that promote increased endurance, muscle growth, and fat burning. The chart above is a graphic summary of published research on diet and human endurance conducted since the 1950s.

Comparing the Diets (page 21) illustrates the glycogen-storing potential of three kinds of diets: the current fad high-protein diet, the ordinary American diet, and the Ultimate Ratio. The Ultimate Ratio helps athletes work far longer than the other two diets and it boosts the body's glycogen stores (listed as grams of glycogen per 100 milligrams muscle tissue) almost six times more than a high-protein diet. To a professional athlete, glycogen is like money in the bank, enabling him or her to draw on those reserves in prolonged activity.

Excess protein drives calcium, potassium, and other minerals out of the body. High-protein diets force the kidneys to excrete urea, a toxic byproduct of protein metabolism. The kidneys must neutralize acids in the urine that are produced as a person digests meat. To buffer these acids, bones must surrender their structural minerals. High-protein diets also force cells to lose potassium, a mineral required for a healthy heartbeat and a properly functioning nervous system. Studies have determined that for each additional gram of protein you eat beyond what you require each day, your body excretes an additional milligram of calcium. This can take its toll on your skeleton over a lifetime, considering that many people, on average, consume thirty to fifty grams of protein beyond what they require each day. Is it any wonder that so many Americans suffer from osteoporosis, the potentially fatal bone-softening disease? People who consume excess salt (more than 3 grams of sodium per day) also retain less calcium in their bones.

Excess protein dehydrates the body. High-protein diets force the kidneys to work hard to rid the body of nitrogen-related waste products. Water and valuable minerals are lost in the body's attempt to detoxify the metabolic waste products of protein metabolism. Active people who follow fad diets pushing protein and fat run the risk of crippling their stamina because of dehydration.

Excess protein causes chronic joint inflammation. Those poor misguided bodybuilders at my local gym. They wolf down steak-and-egg diets and mega-protein sports supplements in a reckless effort to bulk up. The only thing they're going to increase is the amount of inflammatory byproducts of fatty food metabolism that irritate joints and chew up cartilage.

WHY HIGH-PROTEIN DIETS CAME BACK INTO FASHION

The recent glut of protein-pushing diet books appeals primarily to millions of relatively sedentary Americans who got fat while trying to follow a low-fat, high-carbohydrate diet. Government studies reveal that people who thought they were eating a low-fat diet were actually eating more fat and calories than they'd previously eaten. Because they increased their caloric intake more than they increased their fat intake, the percentage of daily fat calories they consumed fell slightly. These people thought they were eating a low-fat, high-carbohydrate diet when, in fact, they were eating far too much fat and sugar for optimal health and fitness. Moreover, they were spending more time in front of computers and TV sets and less time at the gym. Millions of these sedentary Americans who had fooled themselves into thinking that eating a bag of fat-free Snackwell cookies qualified them as being on a low-fat diet were ready to be seduced with the irresistible promises made by the protein pushers.

How did the protein pushers convince Americans to jump on the high-protein bandwagon? First, they promised that people could eat the high-fat foods they already loved, including hamburgers, hot dogs, BBQ ribs, pastrami, lamb, steak, prime rib, and cheese. Second, they promised that, by doing so, people would lose weight and never feel hungry. Third, they promised permanent weight loss. It sounded too good to be true. All people had to do was to keep eating their favorite fatty foods while cutting back on carbohydrates.

The protein pushers had their scapegoat: carbohydrates. And they had millions of frustrated dieters looking for a quick fix to their dietary woes and frustrations. The message was clear: Carbohydrates were the real gremlins that kept people from reaching their perfect weight. That message appealed to dieters who had disciplined themselves to eat an unsatisfying smorgasbord of fat-free salad dressings, fat-free cookies, fat-free muffins, fat-free cakes, and fat-free snack chips in addition to a reasonably large amount of fatty foods. Predictably, these people saw their weight and triglycerides (blood fats) climb instead of fall.

Most high-protein/high-fat diets promise to satisfy our fat cravings and our desire to be slender. Unfortunately, the two are incompatible. It is true that when you curtail carbohydrate consumption, your body temporarily responds in protest with a biochemical chain reaction that suppresses your appetite and leads to weight loss. Of course, that's not all that happens.

KETOSIS: AN UNBALANCED WAY TO BURN FAT

What happens when you limit your intake of carbohydrates on a high-protein diet?

Within a day, your body uses up all of the sugar stored as glycogen in your muscles and liver. Now there are only two fuels left: fat, which is stored in primarily in adipose tissue and around vital organs, and protein, found primarily in muscle tissue. Since your brain ordinarily burns sugar (glucose) as its fuel, which it gets from the carbohydrates you eat or store as glycogen, your body begins to break down muscle protein and convert it into sugar.

To combat the wasting of muscle tissue, the body enlists the liver's help to convert stored fat into ketones (incompletely burned fatty acids), which the brain can use for fuel in place of glucose. Now the body begins to pull out fatty acids from fat cells as it converts them to ketones so that the brain can use them for energy. The resulting condition, called ketosis, is actually the brain's form of crisis management—an emergency measure that helps preserve muscle tissue and vital organs from losing too much protein. Of course, the brain prefers glucose, not ketones, and so people who eat high-protein/low-carbohydrate diets may find they become irritable and a bit foggy when they begin a high-protein/low-fat diet. You know when someone is in ketosis because their breath carries a distinctively unpleasant chemical smell.

The brain also needs to protect itself against the glut of ammonia that results from the metabolism of all that excess protein. Because this protein waste product is so highly toxic, the brain has developed a damage control mechanism to protect itself. The brain detoxifies ammonia molecules by converting them to glutamine. The glutamine is then shuttled to the kidneys, where it is broken down to glutamate and ammonia. There the ammonia is converted to the final product of protein metabolism, urea. As you've already learned, excess ammonia and urea can upset the body's delicate acid-base balance, forcing bones and muscle tissue to surrender vital minerals and water.

THE CAVEMAN THEORY

Humans evolved on a mixed diet of vegetable and animal foods. Prehistoric fossil evidence leaves no doubt of this. Indeed, the structure of the human digestive tract reveals that it is well equipped to handle both types of foods. Some protein pushers like to point out that cave dwellers ate a lot of meat along with root vegetables, seeds, nuts, berries, and other fruits. This is their favorite evolutionary argument for promoting high intakes of animal protein foods. They don't tell you why this is not such a good idea for people today. I will:

Cave dwellers lived on the brink of starvation. The earliest humans subsisted on a low-calorie diet and burned a tremendous amount of calories while hunting prey and gathering root vegetables, seeds, and berries. Laboratory experiments involving controlled starvation in a variety of animal species reveal that very low-calorie subsistence diets and a good deal of exercise (essentially a hunter-gather lifestyle) extend life expectancy and reduce the risk of diet-related diseases. It doesn't matter if lab animals eat a high- or low-protein diet. They'll live longer because of caloric restriction as long as they receive an adequate amount of such nutrients as vitamins and minerals. But who could live on the brink of starvation today? And that's what you'd have to do in order to subsist on a prehistoric cave dweller's diet.

The meat was healthier. Our prehistoric forbears ate meat that contained a healthier fat profile than supermarket meat. Prehistoric animal flesh was also much lower in total fat. So prehistoric people ate a unique, lower-fat diet that cannot be replicated today by eating commercially raised beef, pork, and other meats.

Ketosis helped cave dwellers survive. Fortunately for cave dwellers, the human body goes into a state of ketosis when meat is plentiful and carbohydrate foods are scarce. Since ketosis keeps hunger at bay, cavemen could concentrate on tracking down their dinner without feeling hungry. Ketosis also kept their brains from starving due to lack of glucose until they could find carbohydrate-rich foods. Two hundred thousand years ago, ketosis worked as a survival mechanism. Today, for millions of sedentary Americans, ketosis spells dietary disaster.

The Ketosis Diet Deception

During the early stages of a high-protein/low-carbohydrate diet, the majority of weight comes off rapidly in the form of water and glycogen—not as fat. Three grams of vital water are lost along with every gram of glycogen. During the first week of ketosis, a man can lose almost all of the glycogen stored in his liver and muscles (about 300 g in the liver and about 1,500 g in the muscles). Let's assume he loses a little more than half his total glycogen (1,000 g). We can calculate his weight loss due to water and glycogen:

Water loss: 3 times the weight of lost glycogen (1,000 g):　　3,000 g
Glycogen loss: (200 g from the liver, 800 g from muscles):　　1,000 g
Total weight loss:　　4,000 g

4,000 g = 9 lb of weight loss—none of which represents any fat!

Is it any wonder that people are initially impressed with the results of a high-protein weight-loss diet? All the water and glycogen comes back when carbohydrate intake returns to normal, as it inevitably does.

KETOSIS—AN UNHEALTHY DIET STRATEGY

Some protein pushers use ketosis to induce suppression of appetite. Ketosis will continue as long as you have fat stored in your tissues, provided you keep your carbohydrate intake very low. But the minute you start eating a reasonable amount of carbohydrate-rich foods, your body jumps for joy, bio-chemically speaking, and the liver stops producing ketones. At that point, ketosis is over, and with the end of ketosis, your appetite returns—with a vengeance.

During the first few days on a high-protein/low-carbohydrate diet, your body will use up its glycogen reserves—the last molecules of sugar stored in your liver and muscles. Glycogen holds three times its weight in water, so the burning of these glycogen stores quickly dehydrates the body, which accounts for much of the immediate weight loss.

Over the next several days, the body goes into a state of ketosis, which suppresses appetite. A person in ketosis can subsist on 800 calories a day and not feel overly hungry. Many high-protein dieters feel empowered by being able to get by on so few calories. They feel in control of their eating for the first time. It is this feeling of power over one's natural urge to eat that appeals, at the outset, to so many people. So weight loss—first from water, then from both water and fat—continues for several weeks.

In the short run, a high-protein diet delivers all that its architects promise: weight loss and loss of appetite. But there's a fly in the beef stew, so to speak: At some point, the weight loss slows and carbohydrate cravings inevitably return. And when the cravings come back, so does your appetite and your "lost" body fat. More important, a high-protein/high-fat diet sets the stage for chronic, degenerative diseases. That is the tragedy of such diets. We already know they don't lead to permanent weight loss for most people, but they could lead to permanent disability—or worse. The high-protein animal foods promoted by these diets contain no disease-fighting phytonutrients and they are devoid of fiber.

In my nutritional practice, I meet many people who are aware of the long-term health risks of eating a high-protein diet yet try to live on it anyway. They understand that they are consuming a diet that might lead them directly to disease, but they think they will be the exception to the rule—that they will beat the odds and remain healthy despite volumes of published scientific evidence to the contrary. Others fool themselves into thinking they can use such a diet for its short-term benefit—weight loss—and then chuck it before they suffer serious health consequences. What they don't realize is that there are short-term consequences to such diets as well.

High-protein/high-fat weight-loss diets can increase the risk of suffering from kidney stones, gout, gallstones, and dizziness. By the time high-protein aficionados finally realize that they can't live comfortably forever on a high protein/high-fat, low-carbohydrate diet, they have a great deal of trouble switching to a lower-fat, phytonutrient-based diet because they've cultivated a taste for rich, fatty foods.

THE WRONG KIND OF CARBS

Once a person who has been starving for carbohydrates on a high-protein diet starts to eat cookies, pastries, muffins, and other processed and fat-laden carbohydrate foods, nearly all of the fat in these foods is absorbed and immediately stored by the body. The processing and refining of these foods alter the structure of carbohydrate molecules, making them easier to absorb. These processes also remove the fiber and water, leaving behind more concentrated calories.

The body responds to refined carbohydrate foods differently from a minimally processed natural carbohydrate food such as oatmeal. Processing and refining carbohydrates disrupt the molecular architecture of these foods, permitting the sugars in them to be rapidly absorbed into the bloodstream. In doing so, food manufacturers essentially "predigest" the carbohydrates for you by extracting the sugars from the fiber. Unfortunately, they leave behind the worst and discard the best of the food.

Eventually, many people lose their taste for low-carbohydrate cakes, cookies, and snack foods. They begin to crave the real deal. And the real deal comes loaded with plenty of fat (a typical bran muffin can pack 20 grams of fat or more). What happens when you eat such predigested carbohydrate foods? The fat—but not the sugar—is quickly extracted and stored around your stomach. What happens to the sugar? The brain and muscles use it as fuel.

Insulin, the hormone secreted by the pancreas to clear the blood of excess sugar, pours into the bloodstream when you eat protein and carbohydrates. The protein pushers understand this but try to persuade you that high-protein diets are healthier because they produce less of an insulin spike. Overproduction of insulin is unhealthy, but the protein pushers don't tell you that a phytonutrient-rich diet (naturally low in calories and high in complex carbohydrates) will keep insulin levels stable and will prevent the very diseases, including obesity, that are linked to the high-protein/high-fat diets they promote. More important, they don't tell you that calorie for calorie, high-protein/high-fat foods leave you hungrier than phytonutrient-rich carbohydrate foods. In fact, they tell you just the opposite. They couldn't be more incorrect, as you will discover in chapter 3 when I tell you about the Satiety Index.

HEALTH RISKS SURROUNDING HIGH-PROTEIN/HIGH-FAT DIETS

Few people understand the biochemical havoc they create in their bodies when they slug down the bacon-and-eggs-type breakfast promoted by the protein pushers. From a public health perspective, they might as well be drinking slow-acting poison. Lab animals live a significantly shorter life when fed a high-protein diet (see graph page 29). There's every reason to expect that humans do as well. If this sounds a bit extreme, consider the dangers of eating too much protein and fat; then judge for yourself.

Effect of High-Protein Diet on Life Expectancy of Lab Animals

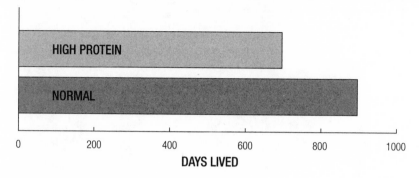

Obesity. As weight increases above a body mass index of about 25, so does risk of premature death.* Being overfat or obese is a risk factor for several types of cancer, heart disease, diabetes, hypertension, and osteoarthritis. Numerous studies link calorically dense diets, high in protein and fat, with obesity.

Cancer. A high-protein/high-fat diet does not contribute to all cancers, but many studies have linked it to colon, prostate, pancreatic, and breast cancer, which together account for nearly 200,000 deaths a year in the United States. Some studies suggest that a high-protein/high-fat diet may play a role in causing lung cancer in nonsmokers (30,000), basal-cell skin cancer (750,000), and malignant melanoma (7,300).

Heart disease. About one American in four suffers some form of heart disease. Cardiovascular disease kills almost 1 million Americans a year; most die from heart attacks. Heart disease results from a process called atherosclerosis, which is directly linked to animal protein foods rich in such artery-bashing compounds as cholesterol, saturated fats, and arachidonic acid.

---

*Body mass index, or BMI, is a measure of body fatness. BMI can be calculated as follows:

1. Multiply your weight in pounds by 703.
2. Multiply your height in inches by itself.
3. Divide the first number by the second.
4. Round to the nearest whole number

The result is your BMI. BMI is not always an accurate measure of body fatness for body builders, the sedentary elderly, and those who are pregnant or nursing.

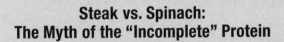

Steak vs. Spinach: The Myth of the "Incomplete" Protein

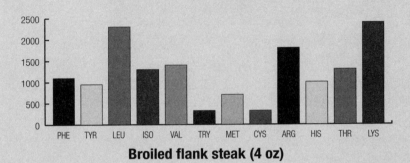

Broiled flank steak (4 oz)

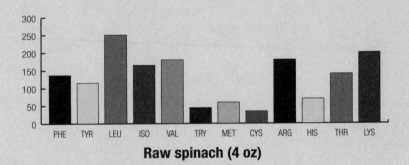

Raw spinach (4 oz)

These two graphs illustrate that spinach contains a nearly identical pattern of all essential amino acids found in beef, clearly dispelling the myth that vegetable protein is somehow "incomplete" and animal protein is "complete." Ounce for ounce, vegetable foods do contain less total protein than animal flesh: spinach and flank steak both contain 40 percent of their calories as protein. Even an Olympic bodybuilder can easily meet his or her protein needs by eating protein-dense legumes and soy foods over the course of a day. Consuming all essential amino acids within a single day (and not within a single meal, as many diet experts mistakenly believe) is sufficient to meet human protein requirements.

PHE = PHENYLALANINE   MET = METHIONINE
TYR = TYROSINE   CYS = CYSTEINE
LEU = LEUCINE   ARG = ARGININE
ISO = ISOLEUCINE   HIS = HISTIDINE
VAL = VALINE   THR = THREONINE
TRY = TRYPTOPHAN   LYS = LYSINE

Although heart disease generally strikes after age forty in men and after menopause in women, arterial damage begins in childhood. Studies reveal that nearly every child in the United States has atherosclerotic plaques in their aortas, the body's largest artery.

High blood pressure (hypertension). Hypertension is a major risk factor for heart disease and stroke (stroke is the nation's third leading cause of death behind heart attacks and cancer, claiming 144,000 lives a year). A high-protein/high-fat diet contributes to this condition because it usually causes obesity and affects the hormones responsible for elevating blood pressure. As weight increases, the heart must work harder to pump blood through extra adipose tissue. As the heart's effort increases, so does blood pressure.

Diabetes. Over 15 million Americans have adult-onset diabetes (250,000 deaths a year). The disease involves an inability to metabolize blood sugar because the body has become insensitive to the pancreatic hormone, insulin.

THE "INCOMPLETE" PROTEIN MYTH

If you had to, you could get all the protein you need by eating spinach or even white bread. Surprised? Hospital dietitians and protein-pushing diet book authors first scowl, then howl with laughter when I point this out. Before you shake your head in disbelief, examine the graph Steak vs. Spinach on page 30. It reveals that spinach contains all the essential amino acids in nearly the same ratio as found in beef. Popeye was right after all.

Professional athletes, trainers, and coaches struggle with this revelation as well. Long-standing myths die hard, especially when they are perpetuated in popular diet books and medical and nutritional textbooks. Read my lips:

There are no "incomplete" protein natural foods.

The notion that foods contain incomplete protein is deeply ingrained in the national psyche. Each year, in a misguided attempt to get "complete" protein, Americans on average consume one and a half times their body weight in red meat, twice their weight in dairy products, and half their weight in chicken and turkey, not to mention 250 eggs each year! With this bounty of animal protein comes an abundance of saturated fat, cholesterol, and arachidonic acid (linked to cardiovascular disease, hypertension, cancer, and arthritis). A growing body of evidence clearly reveals that the real price of all this "complete" animal protein is obesity, disease, disability, and death.

Have you ever stopped to wonder how all that "complete" protein got into the meat, milk, fowl, and eggs? It all came from *carbohydrates*—grains and grasses consumed by steers, cows, and hens. A gorilla doesn't need to eat steak and eggs to grow large and powerful muscles. You don't either.

It should be clear by now that it is almost impossible to eat a protein-deficient diet even if you are a total vegetarian. Remember: If your sole source of protein were spinach, you would still be eating a complete protein. Fortunately, you won't have to do that because the Ultimate Ratio includes a delicious variety of "surf-and-turf" protein-dense foods: seafood (a source of healthy omega-3 fatty acids), soy-rich meat replacers (high in cancer-fighting and cholesterol-lowering phytonutrients), and legumes (rich in antioxidants and fiber).

PROTEIN: THE BOTTOM LINE

The truth, plain and simple, is that high-protein/high-fat diets make losers out of winners. Moreover, they put millions of people at an increased risk for serious health problems.

To many athletes, protein is like a religion: they believe in it and hold it sacred. But there is nothing pious about being a protein junkie. Protein junkies blindly believe that a high-protein diet will improve their sports performance, endurance, and help build larger, stronger muscles. In my experience, no amount of reason or scientific proof can persuade them to recant. Two personal anecdotes illustrate my point:

Former tennis champion John McEnroe, who today is still an excellent competitor on the seniors' tennis circuit and arguably one of the best commentators for televised tennis matches, enjoyed steak and other high-protein/high-fat foods during his professional career. I tried to get John to embrace the Ultimate Ratio, but he simply wasn't interested in changing his diet. He had been taught that high-protein foods were good for athletes, so why should he switch to another type of diet? After all, he had enjoyed great success due to his natural talent for tennis and extraordinary hand-eye coordination. But natural talent can take an athlete only so far. John found this out when he started losing to another talented player, Ivan Lendl. John knew that Ivan's meteoric rise to number one in the world was fueled by the Ultimate Ratio (often referred to on the professional tennis tour as "the Haas diet"). When a reporter asked John if he was on the Haas diet, he retorted in protest, "I'm on the Haägen-Dazs diet!"

•

In 1981, Jim Fixx, a well-known running enthusiast and best-selling author on the subject, asked me to evaluate his blood chemistry profile from a recent physical. His blood cholesterol level was quite elevated—around 275 mg. I told Jim that he was a high-risk candidate for a heart attack, not only because of his elevated cholesterol, but also because his father had died prematurely of heart disease *and* because he exercised so vigorously. Fixx, like the medical doctors who wrote for popular running magazines at the time, believed that jogging would protect him against heart disease. He was able to keep his weight under control with high-mileage running each week. Jim was unaware that exercise and a high-protein diet make a deadly duo because they increase, not lower, the risk of suffering a heart attack. The day I had lunch with Jim, he ate two large servings of roast beef with gravy. I implored Jim to embrace the Ultimate Ratio to get his blood cholesterol below 150 mg and reduce his risk of sudden death. Jim felt that his diet needed to be high in protein and pointed out that his doctor never mentioned going on a cholesterol-reducing diet. So Jim politely demurred my request. Not long after we spoke, Jim dropped dead of a massive heart attack while he was doing the very thing he was certain would protect him—jogging.

So there you have it. Two stories of fine athletes who refused to give up their high-protein diets. In one case, I believe it detracted from a great athlete's success and career longevity. In the other case, it prematurely ended a life. The lesson to be learned is clear: Get out of the high-protein danger zone and into the winner's circle—with the Ultimate Ratio.

3

EAT TO LOSE

PRINCIPLES OF PERMANENT FAT LOSS

I suspect that Oprah Winfrey would love to fit into her Calvins again—the jeans she proudly wore the day she modeled her newly slimmed body for the millions of fans of her TV show. Oprah used a liquid protein diet—a dangerous way to lose weight even while under a physician's care—to shed the equivalent in body weight of an eight-year-old child. She looked fit, svelte, and healthy. A Calvin-clad Oprah made millions believe that their weight-loss dreams could come true.

Sadly—but quite predictably—Oprah started regaining weight after she abandoned her liquid meals in favor of solid foods. No one could or should live on such a rigorous liquid diet indefinitely. Within months, the weight started creeping back. Oprah ballooned up to 225 pounds and couldn't regain her Calvinesque figure despite adherence to a low-fat diet as detailed in her best-selling cookbook, *In the Kitchen with Rosie* (Rosie Daley and Oprah Winfrey).

Gaining but undaunted, Oprah hired a personal trainer and began a rigorous program of long-distance running (at one point she jogged as much as fifty miles a week), even getting fit enough to complete a marathon. Oprah got down to 150 pounds and the weight stayed off as long as she stuck to her demanding workout routine. Oprah was so happy with her jogging-induced weight loss that she wrote a book about exercise—*Make the Connection*—with trainer Bob Greene.

Eventually, as Oprah's mileage went down, her weight went up. Oprah learned that lifestyle extremes—liquid protein diets, very low-fat diets, and marathon running—work only as long as you stick with them. For Oprah and most people, such extremes are impractical if not impossible to maintain. And Oprah may have an additional strike against her: As an African-American woman, she most likely has a lower metabolic rate than that of nonblack women.

It's inspirational when a national role model like Oprah Winfrey demonstrates that self-discipline, diet, and exercise can help reverse a lifelong weight problem. But each year, 90 million Americans follow some form of weight loss scheme; like Oprah, most of them fail to prevent their hard-lost pounds from creeping back. If Oprah—with the advantage of having a personal chef and fitness trainer on call seven days a week—can't permanently maintain her ideal weight, do you really think you have a fighting chance to do any better?

You bet you do—with the Ultimate Ratio. First, I'll tell you why Oprah and millions of American dieters made the wrong connection. Then I'll show you how to make the right one.

WHY OPRAH'S VERY LOW-FAT DIET DIDN'T WORK

Like millions of Oprah fans, I enjoyed watching her wheel out that wagon full of lard—a metaphor for the eighty pounds of body fat she lost while on her high-protein liquid diet. I was even happier when she recognized the grave health risks of such a diet and switched to a very low-fat, high-carbohydrate diet. But even at that moment, I was 95 percent certain Oprah would put the weight back on. How was I so sure? After years of clinical experience and research, I had discovered the truth about *permanent* weight loss—and, with all due respect, whoever advised Oprah to embrace her very low-fat diet obviously hadn't. The Japanese "experience" illustrates why Oprah was doomed from the day she started her very low-fat diet.

VERY LOW-FAT DIETS: THE JAPANESE EXPERIENCE

For centuries, native Japanese have ranked first in the world in longevity. They have also enjoyed very low rates of mortality from cancer and heart disease. Their diet—based primarily on seafood, rice, vegetables, soy foods, and fruits—is naturally high in carbohydrates and very low in fat (6–10 percent) and calories. The phytonutrients in traditional Japanese foods are so powerful that, despite the widespread use of tobacco, Japanese smokers have relatively low rates of lung cancer and heart disease compared to smokers in the United States. Japanese women enjoy a breast cancer rate five times lower than that of American women.

Ah, you think, the Japanese probably have some type of genetic protection against the diseases that stalk most Americans. Such is not the case. When native Japanese migrate to Hawaii and the U.S. mainland, their rates of these diet-related diseases go up proportionally. Today, the streets of Tokyo are littered with American fast-food chain restaurants. And many Japanese, having developed a taste for American fast foods, now face a growing epidemic of obesity and other diet-related diseases for the first time in history. Clearly, genetics plays a minor role, if any, in protecting Japanese men and women from the pernicious effects of the American high-fat, animal protein-rich diet.

What did the Japanese experience teach us? It revealed that native Japanese who migrated to the United States traded their slimness for obesity and their excellent health for disease—all for the taste of fat and sugar. Were these people insane? No, they did nothing more than follow their genetically programmed food preferences—just as nature intended. When they were presented, for the first time, with a smorgasbord of fast foods loaded with fat and sugar, not to mention huge restaurant portions—their preference for the taste of fat and sugar won out over self-discipline. It's a vicious cycle, because eating fat and sugar makes you hungrier for more fat and sugar.

VERY LOW-FAT DIETS CAN'T FIGHT FAT CRAVINGS

The basic diet chemistry of Oprah's very low-fat diet is quite similar to that found in the native Japanese diet. The Japanese who came to the United States couldn't resist giving up a diet that kept them slender and healthy for one that made them fat and sick—so we know that type of diet probably isn't one that will help Oprah—or you—fight fat cravings any better. What about popular very low-fat diets that limit fat intake to no more than 10 percent of total calories? Will those eating plans help you achieve permanent fat loss?

It's not likely. We already know that many Japanese themselves can't stay on this type of diet when they move to the land where burger is king and dairy is queen. While Americanized versions of a 10 percent-fat diet earn high marks for helping to reduce the amount of arterial plaque buildup in some people, they score rather low marks for taste satisfaction. Only a highly motivated person (perhaps one with heart disease) or a self-disciplined person (one of the lucky few who can lose weight and keep it off on *any* weight-loss diet) will stay with these relatively bland regimens for a lifetime.

Let's review what we've learned about the diets discussed thus far:

1. Oprah couldn't maintain the discipline to stick with a very low-fat (10 percent) diet.
2. Japanese natives who migrate to the United States abandon their very low-fat (10 percent) diet for fatty American fast foods and convenience foods.
3. Very low-fat (10 percent) diets don't please most American palates or satisfy the inborn preference and culturally conditioned desire for the taste and mouth feel of fat.
4. High-protein/high-fat diets appeal to our taste for fat. But these diets can lead us to serious health problems and they tend to stimulate carbohydrate cravings in the long run so they won't help most people achieve permanent weight loss.
5. The ordinary American diet causes obesity and diet-related diseases.

None of these diets leads the majority of people who try them to permanent fat loss. Is there any diet strategy that can satisfy our fat cravings, promote optimal health and fitness, and help us achieve lifetime slenderness and optimal health? Yes—the Ultimate Ratio.

THE ULTIMATE RATIO PRINCIPLES OF PERMANENT FAT LOSS

If you learned everything you know about dieting from magazine articles, friends, fad diet books, and TV informercials, you have most likely been misinformed about permanent weight loss. What you usually get from these sources is more fiction than fact.

If you want to achieve permanent fat loss and muscular fitness, you need two things: accurate information and the motivation or desire to use that information. The Ultimate Ratio provides you with a scientifically sound means to redesign your body from the inside out. You can achieve your perfect weight with the Ultimate Ratio. But *you* must supply the desire and motivation to do so.

The basis for a lifetime of slimness can be found in these three Ultimate Ratio Principles for Permanent Fat Loss:

1. Carbohydrates and protein warm you up and slim you down.
2. No matter where your body fat is located, it all comes from the same source: dietary fat.
3. Functional foods and drinks provide the diet chemistry and taste satisfaction that make permanent fat loss possible for millions of people—especially for those who find it difficult to give up fatty meats or their favorite fast foods.

1. Carbohydrates and protein warm you up and slim you down. Research has proved that the body produces considerably more heat when it metabolizes carbohydrates and protein rather than fats. Anything that heats the body—including exercise, spicy foods, warm baths and showers, warm weather, and even fever—promotes the loss of body fat. An area of the brain known as the hypothalamus regulates your body temperature and hunger. The hypothalamus detects changes in body temperature, monitors blood sugar level and the hormones that control it, and keeps track of the glycogen level stored in your body's muscles and liver. The hypothalamus helps regulate body temperature by increasing or decreasing appetite. When you are hot, appetite wanes. Should you get cold, your appetite increases.

2. No matter where your body fat is located, it all comes from the same source: dietary fat. Under normal conditions, your body will not convert carbohydrate and protein to body fat. *Only the fat in your foods will be stored directly as body fat.* You need some fat in your diet for flavor, texture, and good health. The Ultimate Ratio encourages the use of healthy fats found in olive oil, soy foods, soy-based mayonnaise, and such seafood as salmon, tuna, and shellfish. The composition of stored fat in your body is similar to the fat in your diet and can dramatically affect your health and fitness. People in Mediterranean countries, who derive most of their fats from olive oil and seafood, and Asians, who eat a lot of soy foods and seafood, have the healthiest fats stored in their bodies. These two groups are also among the longest-lived people on earth. The Ultimate Ratio emphasizes these friendly fats above all others.

3. Functional foods and drinks make permanent fat loss possible for millions of people who find it difficult to give up meats or their favorite fast foods. The Ultimate Ratio emphasizes the latest generation of functional foods and beverages that appeal to our culturally conditioned tastes for meats and fast foods. Such functional soy foods as "hamburgers," "hot dogs," "chicken nuggets," "bacon," "sausage," "bologna," and "milk" shakes taste like the real thing but provide *more nutrition for fewer calories.* These low-fat food products, which are sold in most supermarkets and natural foods stores, help satisfy the body's genetically programmed craving for the taste of fat while encouraging muscles to burn away excess body fat. As a result, you get to enjoy the taste of fat and satisfy your appetite with foods that are fun to eat.

GLYCOGEN: YOUR KEY TO PERMANENT FAT LOSS

Glycogen is *your* key to burning fat. Control your body's glycogen levels and you control your ability to stay slim for life.

Glycogen, a chemical complex of sugar molecules strung together in multiple, branched chains, is the way your body stores carbohydrate energy. Whether you eat a bowl of pasta or a banana, you body will store these carbohydrates as glycogen.

Your liver and muscles are the glycogen storage tanks of your body. If you understand a few simple mechanics of how these "tanks" empty and fill, you will understand how and why the Ultimate Ratio can bring you a lifetime of slenderness and peak physical endurance.

Your liver's capacity to store glycogen is far less than that of your muscles, but it serves as an immediate source of carbohydrate whenever you need energy. A man weighing 75 kg might store about 1,800 glycogen calories, with about 1,500 of those calories stored in muscles, the intestines, and the kidneys, and the remaining 300 of those calories stored in the liver. A woman weighing 55 kg may store about 1,200 glycogen calories.

Have you ever wondered why men lose more weight than women while eating the same number of calories and getting the same amount of exercise? The primary reason is that, in general, men have more muscle tissue than women, and muscle burns fat. Another reason is that the more muscle tissue you have, the more glycogen you can store. The more often you empty your glycogen tank, the more the body relies on stored body fat for fuel rather than the carbohydrates you eat.

This sexual inequality can be overcome, in certain instances, with the Ultimate Ratio. A woman who eats according to the Ultimate Ratio can lose more body fat than a man who tries to lose weight on a high-protein/high-fat weight-loss diet. Moreover, studies show that a woman on an Ultimate Ratio diet who enjoys regular exercise stands a greater chance of achieving long-term fat loss than a man who follows a high-protein/low-carbohydrate diet.

If you exercised for at least forty-five minutes today, your body's glycogen reserves will be reduced, which means you have room to store carbohydrate derived from your diet. If you haven't exercised, there will be little room to store any sudden burst of carbohydrate that floods your bloodstream during digestion. The body preferentially burns the excess carbohydrate and shuts down fat burning. This is your first clue as to why people who lose weight and keep it off almost always do some form of regular exercise such as walking.

Let's assume that you haven't exercised and that your glycogen storage tanks are topped off. What will happen to the carbohydrates in your next meal?

You might have gotten the impression that carbohydrate foods, including sugar, can be converted into fat. In fact, sugar is rarely converted to stored fat. The conversion of sugar to fat requires too much energy to make it a useful tool for storing energy in the body. Also, with your liver and muscle glycogen tanks full, there is really no place for the body to store the sugar from your next meal. So it burns most of it to meet the body's energy needs, *at the expense of fat.* Now your fuel mix consists predominantly of sugar. So the fat that ordinarily would have been burned for energy remains in your fat cells, which is exactly what you wanted to avoid. Eating high-carbohydrate foods when your glycogen tank is full essentially throws a bucket of ice water on your body's fat-burning furnace.

Now you know why millions of Americans got progressively fatter during the 1980s and 1990s while trying (but failing) to follow a low-fat, high-carbohydrate diet. They exercised less (which kept their glycogen storage tanks full) and ate more calories (on average, about 300 additional calories per day) and ate more fat. *The truth is that most Americans mistakenly believed they ate a low-fat diet when, in fact, they ate more fat and calories than ever before.*

As Americans began to lose faith in carbohydrates, steak houses—the dieter's *bête noire* of the 1980s and early 1990s—regained their appeal. The popularity of Rush Limbaugh, a radio and TV talk-show host and best-selling author with an appetite for beef and other rich foods, instigated the creation of "Rush rooms" in a number of steak houses across the country, where people would come to celebrate beef while they enjoyed Limbaugh's TV show.* Beef was back—big time.

THE MYTH OF THE GLYCEMIC INDEX

The protein pushers convinced the nation that such high-carbohydrate foods as potatoes, oatmeal, and pasta were the cause of fatness. And to prove their point, they pointed to their favorite piece of propaganda—the *glycemic index.*

Most sports nutritionists, coaches, trainers, and dietitians joined the protein pushers in hailing the glycemic index as a valuable tool for helping people pick the healthiest carbohydrate foods. I would like to cast doubt on the wisdom of all of these health and fitness experts in recommending the glycemic index. I am going to show you why it is a poor guide for helping people select foods to help them curb hunger and lose body fat.

The glycemic index is a table of data that contains the arbitrary numerical ranking of an individual food's ability to raise blood glucose levels relative to a reference carbohydrate. Diabetics use the glycemic index to help them make food choices and construct diets. The theory is that diabetics can better determine how to adjust their glucose-lowering medications by knowing which foods will raise blood sugar faster than others. Such thinking may be misleading, however, as you will see in a moment.

Some protein pushers use the glycemic index as a scare tactic to convince you that a high-carbohydrate diet is unhealthy and inappropriate for weight loss. As I pointed out, the glycemic index only measures the blood glucose-raising effects of a single food. It doesn't work as well for food com-

---

*Recently, Rush Limbaugh gave up beef and other high-protein foods and switched to a low-calorie, high-phytonutrient diet when his physician warned him he was headed for adult-onset diabetes. Rush subsequently lost eighty pounds.

binations and meals. But even when used as intended, *the glycemic index is essentially useless for dieters.* Here's why:

Kiwi fruit and watermelon have a high glycemic index rating—higher than that of a chocolate candy bar. Both are rapidly broken down in the digestive tract and absorbed, but because they are so low in calories and contain negligible amounts of fat, they will not add fat to your body. A small kiwi fruit and a hefty chunk of watermelon each contains only about 50 calories. So it doesn't matter if the carbohydrates in a kiwi or a serving of watermelon are absorbed rapidly. There are simply too few to matter. No one ever got fat eating watermelon or kiwis.

What about potatoes? Those rank high on the glycemic index too. Will eating potatoes make you fat?

A medium potato contains about 105 calories. Recent research has shown that among all foods tested, the ordinary baking potato ranks highest on a more useful index for dieters than the glycemic index—one that the protein pushers don't tell you about. It's called the *satiety* index. This index measures the ability of a single food to satisfy appetite and hunger. Potatoes rank highest, followed by other such "fattening" foods as oatmeal and pasta.

Pasta? Isn't that a refined carbohydrate?

Yes. Pasta is generally made from refined wheat flour and water. Homemade pasta recipes usually call for egg yolks, and therefore I don't recommend them. However, ordinary white pasta is a food you can enjoy (as long as you don't top it off with a high-fat sauce) without worrying about weight gain. Pasta is so filling that most people simply won't be able to eat enough of it to make them fat. And, like potatoes, pasta contains not a speck of cholesterol and is very low in fat.

The protein pushers claim that eating potatoes, oatmeal, and such fruits as bananas and watermelon will make you hungry, fat, and unhealthy. This is food faddism at its worst. Unlike the high-protein animal foods promoted by the protein pushers, these foods contain disease-fighting phytonutrients, fiber, and a much greater ability to effectively suppress hunger.

SCIENCE OVER MYTH: THE SATIETY INDEX

Studies conducted by Dr. Susanne Holt and her colleagues at the University of Sydney reveal the superiority of Ultimate Ratio complex carbohydrate foods over high-protein and high-fat foods in quenching hunger. Holt's research dispels the myth that such foods as potatoes, oatmeal, rice, and fruit make you hungry because they are digested and released into the blood faster than high-protein foods.

Using white bread as a control food (which she arbitrarily assigned a value of 100), Holt asked study participants to score thirty-eight different foods on how effectively each food created feelings of fullness, or satiety. Each participant fasted the night before and then ate a 240-calorie portion of a specific food along with a glass of water. During the next two hours, participants filled out a questionnaire to determine the degree of hunger or satiety they felt. After two hours of no food, they were allowed to eat freely from a wide variety of foods until they felt satisfied. Foods scoring higher than 100 were considered more satisfying than white bread and those scoring under 100 were considered less satisfying.

As a group, fruits ranked at the top, with a satiety index 1.7 times that of white bread, but the highest-ranking food was the very one the protein pushers want you to avoid like the plague: the potato. Other foods that scored high in satiety were oatmeal, pasta, apples, and oranges. The irony is that these foods surpassed the ability of nearly all of the high-protein, high-fat foods the protein pushers recommend to quell hunger.

Now you can understand why none of the protein pushers tell you about Dr. Holt's satiety index. It destroys their fundamental premise that carbohydrate-rich foods make you feel hungry and lead to obesity. In fact, the opposite is true. As Holt observed:

> Fatty foods are not satisfying, even though people expected them to be. We think the reason is that the body sees fat as a fuel which should be used only in emergencies—it stores it in the cells instead of breaking it down for immediate use. Because it doesn't recognize the fat (in food) as energy for immediate use, the body does not tell the brain to cut hunger signals, so we go on wanting more.

Foods scoring highest on the satiety index contain fewer calories per gram than the steak, prime rib, cheese, and other rich foods promoted by the protein pushers. And they contain *no* cholesterol.

Holt recently completed a small study comparing the satisfying power of different breakfasts. She observed:

The Satiety Index

All foods are compared to white bread, ranked as "100." **Boldface** type denotes the foods that provide greatest satiety.

Snacks and Confectionery

Cake 65
Cookies 120
Crackers 127
Croissant 47
Doughnut 68
Jellybeans 118
Mars candy bar 70
Peanuts 84
Popcorn 154

Carbohydrate-Rich Foods

Brown pasta 188
Brown rice 132
French fries 116
Potatoes 323
White bread 100
White pasta 119
White rice 138
Whole-grain bread 157
Yogurt 88

Protein-Rich Foods

Baked beans 168
Beef 176
Cheese 146
Eggs 150
Lentils 133

Breakfast Cereals

All-Bran 151
Honeysmacks 132
Muesli 100
Oatmeal 209
Special K 116

Fruits

Apples 197
Bananas 118
Grapes 162
Oranges 202

Carbohydrates Curb Your Hunger

Potatoes rank highest in satiety, nearly seven times higher than the least-satisfying food, croissants. Whole-grain bread is 57 percent more filling than white bread. High-fat foods normally classified as carbohydrates, such as cakes, cookies, and doughnuts, are among the least filling. Fish is more satisfying, per calorie, than lean beef or chicken, which is one reason why it is the primary animal protein food in the Ultimate Ratio. The other reason is that fish contains EPA and DHA—two fatty acids that promote health and fitness.

Two high-fat breakfasts of fried eggs and bacon and toast or croissants and jam were much less filling than two equal-calorie high-carb breakfasts which were either rapidly digested (cornflakes with sugar and toast and jam) or slowly digested (All-Bran with banana slices, toast and margarine).

So the truth is that the high-fat content of eggs, bacon, and croissants can leave you hungrier than a carbohydrate-rich breakfast—even one that contains sugar and processed breakfast cereal. When it comes to high-protein/high-fat meals, you simply can't fill up without filling out. Holt also noted an important side effect of high-carbohydrate meals:

> The two high-carb breakfasts tended to improve alertness to a greater extent than the two high-fat breakfasts. Also, because the subjects were not completely satisfied by the two high-fat meals, they tended to be grumpy and a bit more aggressive/disappointed.

Now you know one reason why the Ultimate Ratio helps you enjoy maximum mental performance and promotes a mind-body connection. The Ultimate Ratio provides superior nutrition to the experimental high-carbohydrate breakfast used by Holt, but the biochemical principles involved in boosting mental focus, concentration, and mood remain the same. If you want to improve your ability to concentrate, focus, learn, do better on tests, and improve your overall mental performance, eat to think with the Ultimate Ratio.

The glycemic index is essentially useless to eat-to-winners because most of the phytonutrient-rich carbohydrate foods of the Ultimate Ratio are so low in calories. And because these foods are the most filling for the least calories, they force your body to release stored fat to be burned for fuel. Only fat-laden carbohydrate foods that contain concentrated calories—such as muffins, pastries, doughnuts, croissants, and cookies—will make you fat. It's *only* the fat in these foods—not the carbohydrates—that will add fat to your body.

ANATOMY IS NOT DESTINY

The good news is that when you begin to lose body fat, your abdominal fat is the first to disappear, thus the easiest to get rid of. The bad news is that if your buttocks, hips, or thighs are your problem areas, those will be harder to reduce in size. And if you are obese, chances are that you will never be able to get rid of all your excess body fat. Here's why: As you gain weight, your fat cells first increase in size, then in number. Obese people (those with a BMI of 25 or greater) have more fat cells than people who are not obese. No diet, including the Ultimate Ratio, can decrease the number of fat cells. Only liposuction can do that. But you can reduce the amount of fat stored in those cells and thus the size of the cells, so you can still become thinner and healthier on the Ultimate Ratio.

THE ULTIMATE RATIO "200" RULE

It doesn't matter if you take a walk, climb some stairs, mow the lawn, play a round of golf, or run a marathon. As long as you move enough to burn off 200 extra *glycogen calories* each day and eat according to the Ultimate Ratio, you will burn off excess body fat. The plan works like magic, but it's nothing more than simple biochemistry. Why haven't you been told this before? Most diet "experts" have failed to put all the pieces of the weight-loss puzzle together. And without all the pieces in place, they couldn't see full picture. But now *you* can. As a rule of thumb, assume that half of the calories you burn during physical activity or exercise consist of glycogen calories. The other half of the calories you burn come from fat. So when you have burned approximately 400 total calories, at least half of those will have come from glycogen.

THE CALORIE MYTH

Many diet experts will tell you that exercise is not a very efficient way to lose weight. They point out that you have to burn 3,500 calories to lose a pound of fat and they tell you you'll have to walk 35 miles to accomplish this. As it turns out, both statements are inaccurate. These "experts" aren't such experts after all. Here's why:

1. You'd have to walk *70 miles* to burn off a pound of body fat—not 35 miles as the experts claim. The reason is quite simple. On average, most people burn a fuel mixture of about 50 percent fat and 50 percent carbohydrate at rest. Depending on the type of exercise you do—aerobic or anaerobic—and amount of time you spend exercising, and the diet you eat, this mixture will vary. But as a rule of thumb, you can use the 50:50 ratio to calculate that

Calories Burned during Selected Activities*
Your Goal: Burn 200 Glycogen Calories Each Day

Activity	Calories per hour	Glycogen calories per hour
Running 10 mph (6-min miles)	1,200	600
Jogging 5.5 mph (11-min miles)	700	350
Cross-country skiing	700	350
Bicycling 12 mph	400	200
Bicycling 6 mph	220	110
Swimming 25 yards/min	250	125
Swimming 50 yards/min	500	250
Tennis—singles	400	200
Walking 2 mph (30-min miles)	220	110
Walking 3 mph (20-min miles)	300	150
Walking 4.5 mph (13.3-min miles)	420	210

*All values are appropriate. Most people will probably burn more glycogen calories than these figures indicate.

the practical caloric cost of burning a pound of body fat is actually closer to 7,000 calories than to 3,500 calories:

1. Walking 1 mile burns 100 calories (50 fat calories + 50 carbohydrate calories).
2. 3,500 calories (usable calories in 1 pound of fat) ÷ 50 fat calories burned/1 mile = 70 miles

2. While this seems to support the argument that exercise is not an efficient way to lose weight, it actually upholds my contention that daily exercise is essential to permanent fat loss. Why? Because burning 50 percent or more of your calories from glycogen allows you meet your daily 200-glycogen calorie goal in just a one-hour walk or its equivalent (most people will probably achieve this within 45 minutes). At the end of that walk, you will also have burned close to 200 fat calories from your stomach, butt, and thighs to boot! I'd call that worthwhile effort. And any activity you do beyond walking is icing on the cake, so to speak.

3. Evidence for the importance of emptying your glycogen tanks with exercise each day comes from laboratories the world over. When researchers allow unexercised lab animals to eat at will from a selection of high-fat and low-fat foods, the animals consume over 50 percent more calories from fat

Calories: Where Do They Go?

Almost all weight-loss experts tell you that all calories, regardless of their source, add fat to your body. This is misleading and inaccurate, as this illustrative example points out.

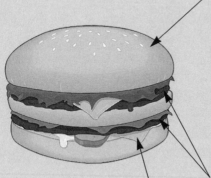

CARBOHYDRATE CALORIES

Used for energy and glycogen:
- The body burns carbohydrates immediately for energy or stores them in the liver and muscles as glycogen.
- Eating carbohydrate calories will not make you fat, but eating too many carbohydrate calories will shut down fat burning and prevent you from losing weight.

PROTEIN CALORIES

Used for growth, maintenance, and energy:
- The body uses protein for growth and maintenance. It also uses muscle protein for energy during exercise if carbohydrates are in short supply.
- Eating excessive protein calories will increase your body's production of the waste products ammonia and urea, which can dehydrate the body and deplete bones of calcium and other minerals.

FAT CALORIES

Stored immediately as body fat:
- The body stores all fats and oils in foods and beverages directly and immediately as body fat.
- Fats and oils in foods are never burned immediately as energy. These are the calories that add inches to your stomach, hips, butt, thighs, and upper arms.

ALL CALORIES ARE NOT EQUAL

Diet "experts" mistakenly believe that the body treats all calories equally, which is not the case. Only the calories from fats and oils in the foods you eat are stored immediately and directly as fat and not burned as energy. The phytonutrient-rich protein and carbohydrate foods of the Ultimate Ratio (e.g., soy foods, legumes, vegetables, and whole grains) will keep you slim for life and promote peak mental and physical fitness.

than do exercised animals. So we know that exercise blunts the desire to consume fat.

4. Exercise plays an essential role in getting you to lose excess body fat permanently. You already know this because you've seen that you have to partially empty your glycogen storage tanks each day to burn off excess body fat and keep it off. Exercise is the safest and most efficient way to do this.

People who don't exercise each day can't store excess carbohydrates, because their muscles stay loaded with glycogen, so the body burns these excess carbohydrates in place of fat. Exercise alone will not keep people slim unless they are lumberjacks or endurance athletes who burn 5,000 to 8,000 calories a day. Eating processed carbohydrates and fat can cause world-class athletes to gain weight, even if they work out every day. Look at most of the top professional tennis stars on the women's tour and you will quickly understand why exercise alone does not guarantee slenderness.

CALORIES DO COUNT—BUT NOT AS DIET "EXPERTS" TELL YOU

It should be clear by now that all calories are not treated equally by the body, despite what many dietitians and physicians proclaim. It all depends on how they are packaged and if your glycogen tank is full or partially empty.

To illustrate this point, let's assume you drive by a fast-food restaurant and in a moment of weakness you go in and eat an order of French fries. What will happen to all of the calories in the fries when you eat them?

If you haven't exercised, the carbohydrate in the potato overwhelms your glycogen storage tanks because they are already full. Your body has no option but to burn the excess carbohydrate for energy immediately and stop burning fat. So your body retains all of its stored fat along with all the fat that soaked into the potato during frying.

The net cost of eating an order of French fries is that you'll keep all the body fat you presently have *plus* an additional 125 calories worth of fat (weighing half an ounce) from the fat in the fries. None of the carbohydrate in the potato is stored as body fat—only the oil used to fry it.

As you can see from this example and the one on page 48, whether you burn calories or store them as fat depends on where the calories come from (fat or carbohydrate) and how much room, if any, you have in your glycogen storage tank. The body resists using its stored fat for energy unless it absolutely has to use it.

Recall what Dr. Susanne Holt, the creator of the satiety index, said about body fat:

> The body sees fat as a fuel which should be used only in emergencies—it stores it in the cells instead of breaking it down for immediate use. Because it doesn't recognize the fat (in food) as energy for immediate use, the body does not tell the brain to cut hunger signals, so we go on wanting more.

So fat in foods does double damage to dieters:

1. Compared to carbohydrate, fat does little to diminish appetite during a meal.
2. Unlike carbohydrate, fat is stored immediately in fat cells rather than being burned for energy.

Of course, you need some fat in your diet for good health and to satisfy your genetic drive for fat and—let's face it—a small amount of fat make foods tasty and fun to eat. That's why the Ultimate Ratio, unlike the very low-fat (10 percent) diets I discussed earlier, permits foods with some added fat and allows you to use a small amount of olive oil and soy-based mayonnaise.

WHY IS STAYING THIN SO IMPORTANT?

One of the largest studies ever to examine the effects of body fat on longevity concluded that thinner is definitely healthier at almost all ages, including well into middle age and beyond.

This study, published in the *New England Journal of Medicine,* was based on American Cancer Society data on over 300,000 men and women followed between 1960 and 1972. Ironically, it was published along with an editorial urging doctors not to push people too hard to lose weight.

The study found that the people who live longest have body mass indexes between 19 and 22, which is much thinner than most Americans. Body mass index, or BMI, is a convenient way of measuring obesity, since it is an easy way to compare the fatness of people of different heights. BMI is a simple ratio: body weight divided by height squared. The study also revealed that mortality increased significantly when people's BMIs reached 25, and it rose even more sharply when BMIs were 30 and over. *Six out of ten American men and five out of ten American women now have BMIs over 25.*

The U.S. government issued weight guidelines in 1990 that were up to twenty pounds heavier than those listed in the Metropolitan Life tables—the bible of healthy weight for height in America since 1959. These tables were already far too generous in their weight allowances. The National Institutes of Health has recently changed its recommended weight guidelines, a change that classified an additional 29 million more Americans as overweight. Under these new guidelines 97 million American adults—some 55 percent of the population—are considered overweight, which places them at risk for adult-onset diabetes, heart disease, and stroke. Many people believe that it's fine to gain some weight as they age, but the truth is that people in their sixties shouldn't weigh any more than those in their thirties. Staying thin is healthiest even as people go through their forties, fifties, and sixties.

Most people have a corrupted visual sense of what constitutes "normal" body weight simply because most other people they see are fat. Tabloid headlines scream from the page when a celebrity "appears" to be too thin. In fact, most of the celebrities targeted by tabloids as being anorexic have simply reached a healthy weight. Because it is so rare that we see someone who has succeeded in ridding their body of excess flab, these celebrities appear to be too thin when in fact they are at an excellent weight.

If we suffered from regular periods of famine, it would be healthy, even desirable, to carry an extra ten pounds of body fat. But we don't, and so the extra ten or twenty or thirty+ pounds most Americans carry pose a health risk, especially when maintained over decades. Recent health surveys reveal that many American women are between thirty to forty pounds over their ideal weight. Many delude themselves into thinking they are thinner than they are by using clothing size as an indicator of fatness. Some clothing manufacturers have quietly made women's garments larger while keeping the numerical size constant. Today's size 8 dress is really the size 10 or 12 dress of twenty-five years ago. Is it any wonder that many women view runway models as anorexic? If anyone has a distorted self-image, it is the overweight woman who regards her own body as being normal and healthy.

DON'T SWALLOW THE "I'M FAT AND I'M PROUD" PHILOSOPHY

The XXXLs of the world are proud, defiant, and tired of stereotypes. They say it's okay to call them fat, as long as you don't make fun of them. At least, that was the message promoted by some 200 mostly female attendees at a recent Million Pound March in Palisades Park in Santa Monica, California. Actually, no one marched anywhere, nor was there any discussion of the two most important elements of fat loss—diet and exercise.

The event, widely reported in the press, has been an ongoing affair since 1972, when the first meeting was held in a New York City delicatessen. The attendees, whose body types range from Roseanne-ish to, well, extra-extra-extra large, sported T-shirts emblazoned with: FAT! SO?, chanted such feel-good-about-ourselves slogans as "We're fat! We're here! Get over it!" and sang affirmation-laced songs: "We're learning to accept ourselves, we're learning to be wise/Our bodies come in different shapes, we don't apologize/Everyone is beautiful and worthy in our eyes/We're proud in every size!" Some extremists even insisted there was no conclusive evidence linking obesity and health problems.

All the hype and hyperbole drove home the three main points the promoters of the annual event—the National Association to Advance Fat Acceptance (NAAFA)—had hoped for:

1. There's no such thing as permanent weight loss.
2. Fat people are fat because of their genetics and not a weakness for Twinkies and Big Macs.
3. The diet industry is a $40 billion annual rip-off.

With all due respect to the NAAFA, these are weak arguments for promoting the acceptance of obesity. The fact remains that obesity is not a good or healthy condition. Granted, there has been too much discrimination, shame, and pain attached to being overweight, and the NAAFA does a good job of sending volunteers into schools to educate youngsters against name-calling and discrimination. But to condone obesity is to ignore the very real health risks that all overly fat people face—premature disability and death from degenerative diseases, not to mention a lifetime of psychological stress and shabby self-image.

Is it really impossible for people with a genetic tendency to gain more weight than other people to reach a healthy weight? The evidence proves they can. We know from historical records that food rationing in Europe and the United States during World War II led to a reduction of obesity and such obesity-related diseases as Type 2 diabetes and hypertension. We all know people who used to be fat who have changed their lifestyles and are now thin. Even the largest person at the Million Pound March is not immune to the slimming and healthy effects of the Ultimate Ratio plus regular physical activity. And that's a message the NAAFA leadership should write on the blackboard a million times.

4

THE ULTIMATE RATIO

PERMANENT FAT LOSS AND WEIGHT MAINTENANCE

During the 1992 Summer Olympics, I was sitting with a group of people watching Jackee Joyner-Kersee leave her competition in the dust. Her magnificent kick at the end of an 800-meter race caused a friend I was sitting with to ask, "Where do you think she gets her incredible energy?" I turned to my friend and gave him an answer he didn't expect: "Jackee (who has recommended *Eat to Win* to all who aspire to athletic greatness) gets her energy from the sun."

Like every athlete in the world—in fact, like everyone in the world—Jackee Joyner-Kersee's muscles require energy from the sun that has been captured and stored in food—but not just any food. Only plants convert the sun's energy directly into usable energy through the process of photosynthesis. This natural miracle, in which plants combine solar energy with carbon dioxide and water, yields *carbohydrates* while it simultaneously releases life-supporting oxygen into the air. Without consuming the sun's energy originally stored in plants, Jackee Joyner-Kersee couldn't move a muscle.

PHYTOCARBOHYDRATES CENTRAL TO THE ULTIMATE RATIO

We humans reverse the process of photosynthesis by breathing in oxygen and converting food back to carbon dioxide, water, and energy, essentially undoing all the work plants have done! You may dine on scrambled eggs and bacon for breakfast and filet mignon for dinner, but every ounce of energy in those foods came not from a hen, pig, or steer but from *plants*.

Specific plant foods—rich in peak-performance phytonutrients and complex carbohydrates—pave the path to Olympic gold and help perpetuate peak athletic performance. Athletes need to extract energy from plants and they need to be able to store it in specific ways and use it more efficiently and effectively than their competitors. One of my jobs as a sports nutritionist is to help athletes accomplish this biochemical feat.

Throughout history, peasants ate healthy diets of phytonutrient-rich carbohydrates while royalty grew fat and diseased eating a diet of refined carbohydrates and animal protein. Today, nearly everyone eats like royalty because refined carbohydrates and high-protein/high-fat foods are affordable and accessible. And that's why most people are fat.

Thanks to the functional foods and beverages of the Ultimate Ratio, you can eat like a king or queen—with all the delicious taste of your favorite foods, including fast foods—but without the health and obesity problems associated with them. No other eating plan offers its unique and powerful diet chemistry. The Ultimate Ratio offers the healthiest and most slimming way to eat for the new century.

THE ULTIMATE RATIO PLANS

There are two forms of the Ultimate Ratio and one of them is right for you:

1. When you want to lose excess body fat and/or build muscle, use the 25-50-25 Fat-Loss Plan.

2. Once you reach your desired weight and muscle mass, you can switch to the 15-60-25 Weight-Maintenance Plan.

• **The 25-50-25 Fat-Loss Plan.** This is the master plan: It contains the *ultimate* ratio of protein-to-carbohydrate-to-fat that will help you burn stored fat from your body while enjoying delicious meals. It will also provide your muscles and brain with the optimal fuel mix to help you go faster, farther, and higher.

• **The 15-60-25 Weight-Maintenance Plan.** This plan will allow you to enjoy additional starches, vegetables, and fruits each day once you reach your perfect weight. Any time you notice a few pounds creeping back (as many people do during holiday eating splurges), you can switch back to the 25-50-25 plan to quickly burn off the excess fat.

The pie charts below and on page 67 depict the technical breakdown and ratio of protein-to-fat-to-carbohydrate of the two Ultimate Ratio plans. When you follow the Ultimate Ratio guidelines in this chapter, your diet will automatically conform to these pie chart totals. If you want to analyze your daily diet and plan Ultimate Ratio meals, recipes, and parties, you can use The Ultimate Ratio Computer Program for Windows, as I do each day. See appendix I, page 221, for details and ordering information.

ULTIMATE RATIO FOOD GROUPS

The easiest way to eat according to both Ultimate Ratio plans is to build each meal around one serving from each of the following groups:

1. **Protein group** (functional foods made from soy protein, seafood, legumes, egg whites, low-fat yogurt, tofu, and Ultimate Ratio functional drink recipes)
2. **Vegetable group** (all vegetables permitted, including Ultimate Ratio functional drinks)

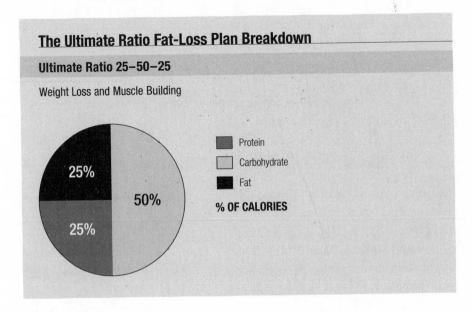

The Ultimate Ratio Fat-Loss Plan Breakdown

Ultimate Ratio 25–50–25

Weight Loss and Muscle Building

25%

50%

25%

- Protein
- Carbohydrate
- Fat

% OF CALORIES

3. Fruit group (all fruits permitted)
4. Fat group (olive oil, canola oil, light or dark sesame oil, soy-based mayonnaise)
5. Starch group (up to two servings each day of oatmeal, brown rice, any whole grain or cereal, whole-grain bread, potato, or any type of eggless pasta)

Optional Groups. In addition to the five main food groups, you may have up to three servings from the **Caffeine group,** one serving three times a week from the **Chocolate group,** and one serving from the **Spirits group** each day.

ADDITIONAL INFORMATION

1. The Ultimate Ratio plan is flexible: As long as you consume the total number of servings per day from each of the four Ultimate Ratio groups, you don't have to eat foods from all four groups in one meal.

2. Use foods and beverages in the **Optional Groups (Caffeine, Chocolate** and **Spirits)** to add variety and flavor to your daily menu. You can enjoy these foods with the confidence that you are consuming disease-fighting phytonutrients even though many fat-loss diets categorize them as "forbidden" foods and beverages.

3. Most Ultimate Ratio functional shakes and cocktail recipes count as multiple food group servings. For example, any shake recipe that contains Soy Cocktail, soy "milk," or provides at least 10 grams of protein per serving counts as one protein serving. If the shake contains fruit or fruit juice, it will count additionally as one or two fruit servings, depending on the amount of fruit used in the recipe. If a drink recipe contains a Twinlab's Phytonutrient Cocktail (e.g., the *Phyto Mary Cocktail*), it counts as two vegetable servings and two fruit servings. Here are three examples:

- One serving of the *Purple Cow* = 2 fruit servings and 1 protein serving.
- One serving of the *Phyto Mary Cocktail* = 2 fruit servings and 2 vegetable servings.
- One serving of the *Orange Genius* = 1 fruit serving and 1 protein serving.

How to Build an Ultimate Ratio Meal

Step 1: Select a Protein-Dense Food

TRADITIONAL
- Seafood (e.g., tuna, salmon, mackerel, shellfish)
- Legumes (peas, beans, lentils)

FUNCTIONAL
- Purple Cow or other soy protein shake
- Soy hamburgers, hot dogs, etc.

Step 2: Select a Vegetable

TRADITIONAL
- Cruciferous (e.g., broccoli, cabbage)
- Carotene (tomato, carrot, yam, squash)
- Sulfur-rich (onion, garlic)

FUNCTIONAL
- Phyto Mary Cocktail (counts as 2 vegetable and fruit servings)

Step 3: Select a Fruit

TRADITIONAL
- Citrus
- Berries
- Pineapple
- Banana
- Cherries
- Blueberries

FUNCTIONAL
- Phyto Mary Cocktail (counts as 2 vegetable and fruit servings)
- Purple Cow shake

Step 4: Select up to 2 Servings per Day of Grains or Cereals

TRADITIONAL
- Whole-grain breads, Pasta.
- Oatmeal
- Brown Rice

FUNCTIONAL
- Any commercially prepared vitamin-fortified whole-grain cereal

Step 5: Select up to 3 Servings per Day of These Fats/Oils

TRADITIONAL
- Olive oil
- Canola oil
- Light or dark sesame oil

FUNCTIONAL
- Nayonaise (soy mayonnaise)
- Fish oil supplement such as MaxEPA

PROTEIN-DENSE FOODS

The Ultimate Ratio emphasizes soy foods and beverages, seafood, and legumes as primary high-quality protein sources. By combining the omega-3 fats, proteins, and phytonutrients found in these foods, your diet will contain an optimal amount of amino acids, energy co-factors, and disease-fighting chemicals in the proper ratio for peak mental and physical performance.

Ultimate Ratio Food Groups and Serving Sizes

Select one serving of your favorite foods from the list below to build an Ultimate Ratio meal. You may substitute any Ultimate Ratio recipe that contains the same primary food (e.g., the **No-Alarm Chili** (page 201) can replace any food from the protein group). Serving sizes are listed in parentheses. Approved functional drink recipes are in **boldface** type. If you must drink alcoholic beverages, limit your intake to the suggested serving size. If you are pregnant or breast-feeding, do not consume alcohol of any kind.

I. PROTEIN GROUP
1 SERVING (4 OZ)

SOY FOODS

Chicken
Ground beef
Hamburger
Hot dogs
SOY DRINKS
Purple Cow (1 serving)
Creamsicle Power Punch
(1 serving)
Thick Chocolate Malted
(1 serving)

FISH

Anchovies
Cod
Grouper
Haddock
Halibut
Mackerel
Salmon
Sardines
Shellfish
Sole
Trout
Tuna

LEGUMES

Beans (½ cup)
Lentils (½ cup)
Peas (½ cup)
Avoid nuts and seeds during fat loss.

DAIRY

Egg substitute
Egg whites (3–4)
Skim milk (1 cup)
Yogurt (non-fat, low-fat; 1 cup)

II. VEGETABLE GROUP
1 SERVING (½ CUP)

Artichokes
Broccoli
Cabbage
Carrots
Cauliflower
Endive
Kale
Onions
Phyto Mary Cocktail (counts as 2 vegetable servings)
Radishes
Squash
Tomatoes
Yams
Zucchini
All other vegetables Avoid avocados and olives during fat loss.

III. FRUIT GROUP
1 SERVING (1 MEDIUM)

All berries (½ cup)
Apples
Bananas
Grapefruit (pink preferred; ½)
Grapes (½ cup)

Kiwi
Mangoes
Melons (all types) (½ cup)
Oranges
Papayas (½ cup)
Phyto Mary Cocktail (counts as 2 fruit servings)
Peaches
Pears
Prunes (4 medium)
Strawberries (½ cup)
All other fruits
Avoid dried fruits during fat loss.

IV. FAT AND OIL GROUP
1 SERVING (1 TEASPOON)

Canola oil
Light or dark sesame oil
Olive oil
Soy-based mayonnaise (Nayonaise)

OPTIONAL GROUPS

STARCH GROUP (up to 2 servings each day)
1 SERVING (½ CUP; 1 SLICE)

Brown rice
Brown rice crackers (9; Hol-Grain brand)
Potatoes (white or sweet: 1 medium)
Whole-grain breads
Whole-grain cereals

Ultimate Ratio Food Groups and Serving Sizes *(cont.)*

CHOCOLATE GROUP (up to 1 serving three times each week)
1 SERVING (½ OZ)
Bittersweet milk chocolate (preferred)

Regular semi-sweet milk chocolate

SPIRITS GROUP
UP TO 1 SERVING EACH DAY

Dark beer (8 oz)
Kahlua (1 oz)
Red wine (3½ oz)
Sake (2½ oz)

Soy Foods. Japanese men, who eat traditional diets rich in soy foods, legumes, and seafood, have a much lower rate of prostate cancer than Americans do. When Japanese men migrate to the United States and adopt a meat-based Western diet, their rate of prostate cancer approaches that of American men. Native Japanese women, who enjoy a breast cancer rate nearly five times lower than American women, suffer higher rates of the disease when they move to the United States and embrace the ordinary American diet.

Soy beverages are an excellent source of disease-fighting phytonutrients. The Ultimate Ratio recommends replacing cow's milk with soy milk whenever possible. Skim milk and fermented skim milk products, such as yogurt and buttermilk, are permitted in small amounts (up to 3 cups per week) and as called for in Ultimate Ratio recipes. In the table on page 61 is a list of Ultimate Ratio recommended functional foods and drinks.

Seafood. Such seafood as salmon, mackerel, sardines, anchovies, and tuna contain omega-3 fatty acids. These fats can help reduce muscle and joint inflammation and reduce the risk of degenerative diseases. Studies have shown that people who eat just one serving of fish each week enjoy reduced risk of cardiovascular disease.

Legumes. The Ultimate Ratio also emphasizes all types of beans, peas, and lentils. Legumes are protein-dense and contain cholesterol-lowering fiber and phytonutrients that can prevent cancer, heart disease, and Type 2 diabetes. Legumes are also a low-fat and cholesterol-free food source of iron and calcium. Dozens of scientific studies have shown that legumes can reduce the risk of plaque buildup in arteries and keep blood sugar level in diabetics.

Ultimate Ratio Recommended Functional Food and Beverage Products

Brand Name	Product Name	Address/Phone/Website
LIGHTLIFE	Smart Deli Meatless Country Ham Style Slices Smart Deli Meatless Roast Turkey Style Slices Smartdogs-✱	P.O. Box 870 Greenfield, MA 01302 1-800-274-6001 Ext. 114 www.lightlife.com
MORNINGSTAR FARMS	Breakfast Patties Breakfast Strips Chik Nuggets ✱ Chik Patties Harvest Burgers Veggie Burgers ✱	Worthington Foods Worthington, OH 43085 614-885-9511
BOCA BURGER	Boca Breakfast Links and Patties Boca Burgers ✱ Ground Boca Burger Recipe ✱ Basics	www.bocaburger.com
NASOYA	Nayonaise	800-229-8639
SOYCO	Lite and Less Grated Parmesan Alternative	Soyco Foods 2441 Viscount Row Orlando, FL 32809 407-855-6600
TWIN LABORATORIES	Choline Cocktail MaxiLIFE Phytonutrient Cocktail MaxiLIFE Soy Cocktail Quix Fix Energy Drink	150 Motor Parkway Suite 210 Hauppage, NY 11788 800-645-5626 www.twinlab.com
YVES VEGGIE CUISINE, INC.	Ground Round (Italian and Regular) Pizza Pepperoni Tofu Wieners Veggie Breakfast Links Canadian Veggie Bacon Veggie Deli Slices	Delta Vancouver, BC Canada V3M 6R9

CHEATING WITH MEAT

Realistically, you or members of your family may want to indulge your taste for beef, pork, lamb, veal, chicken, and turkey—which is fine—as long as you follow these simple guidelines:

1. Consume no more than a 4-ounce portion (about the size of your fist or a deck of cards) per meal. Trim the visible fat from meat and remove the skin from fowl.
2. Limit consumption to two meals (8 ounces total) per week.

Okay—that's pretty simple and easy to follow, isn't it? The guidelines give you some latitude to cheat with meat while following the Ultimate Ratio. They will even allow you and your family to eat at a fast food restaurant occasionally (see Ultimate Ratio Dining Out Guidelines, page 69).

VEGETABLES

The Ultimate Ratio emphasizes vegetable protein from vegetables and soy foods. But not all vegetables are created equal. Some contain more powerful phytonutrients than others, such as those that contain a rich supply of carotenoids, and those known as crucifers, which contain sulfur-based antioxidants.

Carotene/Lycopene-Rich Vegetables. You're probably familiar with two members of the carotene group already—vitamin A, obtained from animal foods, and beta-carotene, the plant form of vitamin A. But there are other members of this family that are equally as important to optimal health, especially lutein, zeaxanthin, and lycopene.

Lycopene quenches the type of free radicals caused by exercise and air pollution. Of all the lycopene-rich foods in our diet, tomato sauce (including ketchup and tomato-based barbecue sauces) contains the highest concentrations of this vitamin. Unlike synthetic beta carotene dietary supplements, which contain no lycopene or any other natural carotenoids, heat-processed tomato products contain a number of free-radical–fighting carotenes. Lutein and zeaxanthin are powerful antioxidants and help protect eyesight.

Tomatoes also contain such additional powerful phytonutrients as p-coumaric acid, chlorogenic acid, alpha carotene, beta carotene, and ascorbic acid. This phytonutrient profile may explain why tomatoes lower the risk of cancers of the prostate and digestive tract and why people who eat a Mediterranean diet enjoy comparatively lower rates of these and other cancers. Carotene-rich foods can also help prevent vision loss due to macular degeneration and poor circulation (a leading cause of blindness in the elderly).

Most people get their carotenoids from carrots, followed by dark-green leafy vegetables, sweet potatoes, oranges, and cantaloupe. I recommend that you consume at least three servings of tomato sauce each week if possible. Tomato sauce is a rich source of the carotenoid lycopene. Lycopene can help protect against heart disease and some types of cancer.

Cruciferous Vegetables. Cancer-fighting cruciferous vegetables prevent estradiol, a potent form of the sex hormone estrogen, from changing normal cell growth to the uncontrolled growth that leads to cancer. In addition, these vegetables direct the body to manufacture enzymes that detoxify chemicals in the environment called xenobiotics (literally "foreign life"). People who consume broccoli and cabbage actually increase the amount of these detoxifying enzymes in their liver, thereby speeding up xenobiotic metabolism and disposing of potential carcinogens. Cruciferous vegetables are important to athletes who compete and train in areas with high levels of air pollution.

STARCHES: WHOLE GRAINS AND CEREALS

Whole-grain breads and cereals contain fiber, a substance that mops up the body's toxic waste and hastens its elimination. Another nutrient, GLA, found in oatmeal, helps lower levels of inflammatory arachidonic acid (AA) in the body.

The fiber found in starches is important to athletes because it helps blunt the rise in blood glucose that can lead to overproduction of insulin and, consequently, hypoglycemia. Most people consume about five to ten grams of fiber each day. Some health experts recommend much higher levels—in the neighborhood of 35 to 40 grams a day.

Oatmeal is the official breakfast cereal of champions of the Ultimate Ratio. It is head and shoulders above all other breakfast cereals because it contains essential fatty acids, disease-fighting phytonutrients, and cholesterol-lowering soluble fiber that also helps maintain stable blood sugar levels.

FRUITS

Citrus fruits play an important role in the Ultimate Ratio because they promote health and fitness. Such citrus fruits as oranges, grapefruit, and lemons contain a number of extremely powerful phytonutrients that can help reduce muscle soreness and damage due to overtraining. Citrus contains potent anti-cancer compounds—so potent, in fact, that a recent study revealed that people who eat citrus fruit daily enjoy more than a tenfold lower cancer risk than those who rarely eat citrus. That's why I recommend you eat at least one citrus fruit each day.

Quercetin is a phytonutrient found in oranges, cranberries, strawberries, apples, and grapes. Quercetin is just one of over 20,000 compounds called *bioflavonoids*. Quercetin is a phytonutrient effective against muscle soreness and muscle damage due to overtraining. Quercetin and other bioflavonoids also help heal damaged capillaries, which supply vital nutrients to muscles.

Dried fruits are highly concentrated in sugar and calories. While they contain important phytonutrients, when you want to lose body fat you should avoid them until you reach your ideal weight.

ADDED FATS AND OILS

With all the health risks associated with high-fat diets, you may be surprised to learn that there are a few fats that actually improve health and fitness. The Ultimate Ratio replaces all added fats and oils in your diet with olive oil, because it contains phytonutrients and fatty acids that promote good health. Extra-virgin olive oil (derived from the first pressing, and the most acidic) is the healthiest type of olive oil because it contains the highest concentration of disease-fighting phytonutrients. Light or extra-light olive oil is a good choice for recipes in which the taste of extra-virgin olive oil would be inappropriate.

When olive oil replaces other fats and oils in your diet, the inflammation potential of your diet decreases, allowing joints and muscles to recover faster and with less damage after vigorous physical activity or injury. Olive oil can also help reduce the risk of heart disease when it supplants the saturated fats and trans-fatty acids (found in meat, milk, butter, and many commercially prepared baked goods) in your diet.

Canola oil, like olive oil, is high in monounsaturates. It contains the omega-3 fatty acid ALA (alpha-linolenic acid). This is the same omega-3 fatty acid found in high concentrations in flaxseed (17 percent by weight) and can also be found in smaller concentrations in walnuts and leafy vegetables. ALA tends to reduce both beneficial and harmful prostaglandins— hormone-like chemicals made by the body that help regulate immunity and control such vital bodily functions as inflammation and healing.

Sesame oil contains monounsaturates in addition to sesamin, a compound that possesses anti-inflammatory and cholesterol-lowering properties. It can also help detoxify carcinogens found in foods and water. You can use this oil on occasion in place of olive oil. Certain Asian dishes, prepared in restaurants or at home, taste better when made with sesame oil.

The other added fat on the Ultimate Ratio plan is soy-based "mayonnaise" (Nasoya's Nayonaise is my first choice). It makes an excellent replacement for real mayonnaise in Ultimate Ratio recipes. It contains no cholesterol, has half the fat of regular mayonnaise, and contains powerful soy isoflavones that lower blood cholesterol levels and reduce the risk of cancer and heart disease.

THE CHOCOLATE FOOD GROUP

Chocolate? On a permanent fat-loss plan? Yes—pure, rich, milk chocolate— light or dark, regular or bittersweet.

Most of my clients are surprised to learn that they can—well—cheat with chocolate and "get away with it," so to speak. The truth is, chocolate is a perfect food with which to cheat because of its healthful properties. Here's why:

- **Chocolate—in the recommended amounts—won't make you fat.** A half-ounce serving of milk chocolate contains only 75 calories.
- **Chocolate contains powerful disease-fighting phytonutrients.** Chocolate contains the same type of phytonutrients found in grapes, tea, and vegetables known to protect against cancer and heart disease.

- **Chocolate contains saturated fats but does not raise serum cholesterol levels.** In fact, a recent study revealed that giving several ounces of chocolate bars per day to young men actually led to a drop in their blood cholesterol levels. The major fatty acid in cocoa butter—stearic acid—is converted to oleic acid, a monounsaturated fatty acid, which does not raise blood cholesterol levels as do saturated fats. Of course, eating too much chocolate is not healthy, so stay within the suggested guidelines. The low-calorie content of one-half ounce of chocolate should pose no health risk to most people.
- **Chocolate is tooth-friendly.** Despite the fact that it contains sugar, chocolate contains phytonutrients that create an unfriendly environment for the type of bacteria that causes dental caries (cavities). Sorry—you still have to brush and floss!
- **Chocolate makes you feel good.** Chocolate can behave as a stimulant in some people, yet exerts a calming effect in others. How chocolate affects you depends on your diet, sleep patterns, gender (it seems to elevate mood in females more than in men, but additional research is needed to confirm this anecdotal observation), and genetics.
- **Chocolate helps you stick to your fat-loss plan.** Indulging in a delicious and healthful treat like chocolate can keep you from feeling deprived while dieting. In my clinical experience, people who rely on chocolate to satisfy their urge to enjoy a tasty treat seem to find it easier to stick with their weight loss plan than those who don't.

Replace These Foods:	With These Foods:
Beef, pork, lamb, fowl	Soy meat replacers
Conventional mayonnaise	Soy "mayonnaise"
Egg yolks	Egg whites
Conventional candy bars	Eat to Win energy bars; Lindt Excellence dark chocolate (70% cocoa)
Ice cream	Frozen fruit bars
Milkshakes	Soy protein shakes
Margarine, full-fat butter	Light butter
Vegetable oils	Olive oil
Full-fat milk, 1%- and 2%-fat milk	Non-fat or 1%-fat soy milk; skim milk
Peanut butter and jelly sandwich	Tuna salad sandwich
Cheese	Soy "Parmesan" cheese

As long as you don't exceed the recommended amount of chocolate per week (one and a half ounces), you will be able to enjoy the taste and health benefits of this unique food product in the Ultimate Ratio plan. Dark bittersweet chocolate contains less sugar and more phytonutrients than regular milk chocolate because of its higher cocoa content.

There are many fine chocolates to pick from, such as Godiva and Lindt brands. I prefer Eat to Win energy bars (of course) and Lindt Excellence dark semi-sweet chocolate made with 70 percent cocoa butter because it has the highest phytonutrient content of any commercial brand of chocolate. If you can't find the 70 percent cocoa version, regular Lindt Excellence will do nicely. Hot cocoa made from pure cocoa powder also contains the same powerful phytonutrients as chocolate. Preparing hot cocoa made with soy milk is a wonderful idea, especially for kids who don't consume enough phytonutrients from vegetables. Note that white chocolate has no phytonutrients because it's not made from cocoa beans.

CONDIMENTS

When it comes to sugar and salt, less is better for everyone. I recommend that you do not use added salt in cooking or at the table. There is no reason to add sugar to foods because of the availability of sugar replacers. My

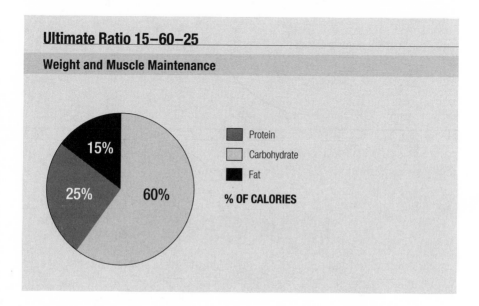

Ultimate Ratio 15–60–25

Weight and Muscle Maintenance

15%
25%
60%

- Protein
- Carbohydrate
- Fat

% OF CALORIES

A 3-Day Sample Menu from the Ultimate Ratio Diet

Meal	Day 1	Day 2	Day 3
Breakfast	• Purple Cow shake (page 167) • ⅓ cup Haas Hummus (page 183) with 6 Hol-Grain Rice Crackers	• Orange Genius shake (page 166)	• Purple Cow shake • Morningstar Farms Harvest Burger (no bun); ketchup
Mid-Morning Snack	• Half a grapefruit	• Apple	• Half a grapefruit
Lunch	• Cup of bean, tomato, and macaroni soup (pasta e fagioli)	• "Meaty" Baked Ziti) (page 205)	Spaghetti with marinara sauce
Mid-Afternoon Snack	• Phyto Mary Cocktail (page 167)	• Phyto Mary Cocktail	• Phyto Mary Cocktail
Dinner	• Big Max Burgers and Special Sauce (pages 186, 181) • Fabulous French Fries (page 193) • ½ cup steamed broccoli with lemon juice • Mixed green salad with balsamic vinaigrette	• Shrimp served over spaghetti with marinara sauce • Mixed green salad with balsamic vinaigrette • ½ cup steamed broccoli with lemon	• Poached Salmon (page 206) • ½ cup steamed Broccoli, carrots, or cauliflower • Baked potato with low-fat sour cream and chives • Mixed green salad with balsamic vinaigrette .
Evening Cheat	• ½ ounce chocolate	• ½ ounce chocolate	• ½ ounce chocolate

Daily percentages of protein, fat, and carbohydrate will vary depending upon portion sizes and foods.

favorite sugar replacer is sucralose, now used in Ocean Spray Lite Style fruit juices. So far, sucralose appears to be the sugar substitute with the least potential for causing side effects. All herbs and spices ordinarily used in cooking are permitted on the Ultimate Ratio plan.

REPLACING PROBLEM FOODS

My experience helping people achieve health, fitness, and permanent fat loss has enabled me to create a short list of foods that you should avoid altogether. Please do not take this list lightly. These foods can upset the diet chemistry of the Ultimate Ratio. Replacing these foods with Ultimate Ratio traditional and functional foods will help ensure your success:

THE 15-60-25 PLAN, ONCE YOU'VE REACHED YOUR GOAL

Once you've achieved your perfect weight and/or desired level of muscular development, you can begin to follow the Ultimate Ratio 15-60-25 plan. This will allow you to maintain your new body weight while enjoying the additional phytonutrients and more of the peak performance foods that helped you achieve your personal health and fitness goals. This plan provides the same amount of protein as the 25-50-25 plan, but because you consume more phytocarbs on this plan, the percentage of daily calories from protein goes down to 15 percent.

Ultimate Ratio Dining Out Guidelines

Burger King: mixed garden salad; Whopper Junior (lettuce, tomato, hold the mayo).

Chinese: grilled tofu; stir-fried mixed vegetables; seafood chow mein; hot and sour soup.

Indian: chicken or shrimp tandoori; nan; raita; basmati rice; lentils.

Italian: any pasta with marinara sauce; chicken cacciatore; pasta e fagioli; shrimp or lobster fra diavolo; minestrone soup; mixed garden salad with low-fat dressing; fresh fruit.

Japanese: kappa maki roll; California roll; tekka maki roll; grilled tofu; mixed salad with miso dressing; shrimp and vegetables; teriyaki salmon; miso soup; *edamame* (steamed fresh soybeans); steamed spinach; cucumbers in vinegar.

Taco Bell and other Mexican restaurants: bean burritos, beef tacos (lettuce, tomato, and no cheese); pinto bean or black bean soup; shrimp or chicken fajitas; grilled salmon or mahi-mahi.

Pizza Hut: thin-crust pizza (made with tomato sauce, half the normal amount of cheese); mixed garden salad with low-fat dressing.

Red Lobster and other seafood restaurants: broiled salmon, tuna, mahi-mahi, or lobster (no melted butter); steamed vegetables, baked potato, salad with low-fat dressing.

Steak house: 4-ounce serving of sirloin steak (split one dinner with another person or take the leftover steak home); broiled chicken breast; broiled salmon; steamed broccoli; mixed garden salad with low-fat dressing.

Wendy's: mixed green salad—chickpeas, carrots, lettuce, red cabbage, and low-fat Italian dressing; baked potato; chili; chicken sandwich with lettuce and tomato (hold the mayo).

The Ultimate Ratio 15-60-25 plan is best suited for people who (1) find they are losing too much body fat on the 25-50-25 plan; (2) would like to add more food volume and variety to their diets.

You will automatically achieve the 15-60-25 maintenance plan when you add the following foods to the Ultimate Ratio 25-50-25 fat-burning/ muscle-building plan:

1. two additional Vegetable group servings;
2. two additional Starch group servings;
3. one additional Fruit group serving;
4. one additional Fat group serving.

Which plan is right for you? Many people prefer to stay with the master 25-50-25 Ultimate Ratio plan, especially those who want to remain on a reduced-calorie diet. Recent research has revealed that subsisting on this type of diet may actually be able to extend life expectancy because it seems to slow the aging process. We already know that it does precisely this in laboratory animals, but no one is yet certain if humans reap the same life-extension benefits. I personally eat this way because I believe it does extend life expectancy by reducing the risk of diet-related diseases and free-radical damage.

Both the 25-50-25 plan and the 15-60-25 plan will help you enjoy excellent health and fitness. Regardless of which plan suits your tastes and personal needs best, you can rest assured that you are following the most scientifically advanced eating plan available.

A CAUTION ABOUT ALCOHOL

Alcohol is a drug, not a food, and as such is limited on the Ultimate Ratio plan. Alcohol intake is directly associated with cancers of the oral cavity, pharynx, esophagus, and larynx, where alcohol acts in concert with smoking to increase the risk. Alcohol consumption has also been linked to breast, colorectal, liver, and pancreatic cancers. A recent comprehensive analysis of studies linking alcohol consumption and breast cancer incidence in women reveals an estimated 25 percent increase in risk for daily alcohol intake equivalent to two drinks. Analysis of data from the largest studies shows that men who drink more than two drinks daily, each containing approximately thirty grams, or one ounce, of alcohol, have twice the risk of developing colon cancer as men who drink less than one quarter of a drink daily.

Is there a positive side to alcohol consumption? The jury is still out. For example, a number of recent studies suggest that men who drink moderately (about two servings of wine, beer, or hard liquor a day) may reduce their risk of heart disease and prostate cancer. I am not convinced that alcohol confers a health advantage to someone who eats according to the Ultimate Ratio and eschews all forms of alcohol.

Wine contains phytonutrients that can help fight cancer and heart disease, but so do grapes and grape juice. These phytonutrients, known as polyphenols, are available in many fruits and vegetables, so there is no need to drink wine or other alcoholic beverages to obtain their health benefits. Chocolate lovers take note: A 1.5-ounce piece of milk chocolate contains the same amount of polyphenol activity as a 5-ounce glass of red wine.

In many people, alcohol can create a cancer-friendly environment that may increase the risk of hormone-sensitive cancers and fuel the growth of precancerous lesions. Alcohol has a toxic effect on many organs, including the liver, kidneys, heart muscle, and bladder.

Just two alcoholic drinks can reduce your heart's work capacity by up to 20 percent for up to twenty-four hours. And alcohol is a potent diuretic— hardly something an athlete wants to deal with in competition.

BUT IF YOU MUST HAVE THAT COCKTAIL . . .

I've worked with many athletes who love beer, wine, and other alcoholic beverages and would never dream of giving them up. Fred Stolle, a Wimbledon champion from Down Under, loved to quaff a pint or two with his mates after a hard day on the courts. Of course, beer is like mother's milk to an Aussie, so when I began working with Fred, I knew there wasn't much chance he'd abstain from alcohol.

After counseling Fred and other athletes who had a fondness for alcoholic beverages, I realized I had to devise a way to combat the pernicious effects of alcohol on the body. After all, alcohol is the closest thing to embalming fluid that we consume. In fact, the liver converts alcohol to formaldehyde during its metabolism. Now you know why we use the term "getting pickled" to denote someone who has had a "few too many." Formaldehyde and other metabolic products of alcohol can adversely affect vision and brain function—the last thing any athlete needs before competition—and then there is the ubiquitous hangover.

I wouldn't want anyone to abstain from the Ultimate Ratio plan because of a preference for alcohol, so I developed a drink based on a functional beverage that not only reduces the pernicious effects alcohol perpetrates on the body, but also mitigates the rather unpleasant morning-after hangover. My adult drinking clients report that my Un-Screwdriver (page 174) contains its own hangover cure!

5

ARE YOUR KIDS FAT OR FIT?

HOW ABOUT *YOU?*

The little victims play!
No sense have they of ills to come,
Nor care beyond today.

—THOMAS GRAY (1716–1771)

"Maybe they're not doing enough in the way of activity. Maybe they
don't have jobs. Maybe they're not doing anything but sitting around
eating."

—JULIA CHILD on why American kids and teens are fat

Fitness clown Richard Simmons wags his finger at the television set.
"It's crazy," he says. "The ads say 'eat, eat, eat!' but show a girl
who's so thin she clearly never eats."

Simmons's beef, clearly, is with the unrealistic message conveyed by
many TV ads that depict a fat-free model enjoying full-fat premium ice
cream. The message is obvious: If she can indulge her taste for frozen cream
and sugar and stay that thin, then so can you. In reality, she probably does a
lot more sweatin' and tonin' than eatin'—a fact not lost on Simmons and a
number of health experts who are understandably annoyed by the incon-
gruity of a slender siren spooning down a carton of Triple Brownie Overload.

Most kids and teens, on average, watch over 10,000 food ads a year on
TV. And I'm not talking about commercials for broccoli. Watching the *Tele-*
tubbies is one thing. Looking like the *Teletubbies*—well, that's a much more

serious matter. American children in the 1990s are the fattest and the least physically active kids in our nation's history. When they play games, it's more often on computers than on baseball fields. The result: Nearly 75 percent of our children are overweight (25 percent are classified as clinically obese) and the President's Council on Physical Fitness and Sports reports that three out of four school-age children have three or more risk factors for heart disease.

Say goodbye to Generation X and say hello to Generation J—J for Junk. Our children are the first crop of truly hard-core junk-food junkies. Gen-J gulps down more sugar-saturated soft drinks, calorific candy bars, sucrose-coated breakfast cereals, and fatty fast foods than any other age group in history. Example: Teenage boys, on average, chug 3⅓ cans of pop each day—that's more than 110 gallons a year; teenage girls guzzle 2⅓ cans daily. Kids today drink twice as much soda as milk, whereas twenty years ago the reverse was true. Today's candy-in-a-can guzzlers make the Pepsi Generation look like teetotalers. And their vegetable of choice: French fries.

THE NEW JEAN-ETICS OF GENERATION J

Our children may start out as tater tots, but they're growing up to be couch potatoes.

Ever since Wendy's out-beefed the Big Mac with their ¾-pound whopper-of-a-burger and two ice cream mavens named Ben & Jerry concocted calorically costly cartons of Chunky Monkey and Chubby Hubby, it's been getting harder for kids to slide into their blue jeans without using a shoehorn. Of course, that's probably why you can't find slim-cut jeans on the shelves of the Gap any more: only jeans the size of camping tents are sold. Today's denims, rechristened with anatomically sensitive terms such as "relaxed fit," "extra baggy," and "wide-leg," are so generously tailored that they contain almost enough extra material for a second pair.

The folks at the Gap are well aware that most American kids and teens have no choice but to buy jumbo-sized jeans. They simply cannot wedge their ample fannies and thighs into the skin-tight designer jeans their parents snugged into just twenty years ago.

All indications are that the trend toward childhood obesity will continue. Actually, it seems to be getting worse. Kids may start as active toddlers, but by the time they enter high school half of the girls and a quarter of the boys don't routinely participate in physical activities. The American social system encourages overeating: Restaurants and food manufacturers compete with one another by offering bigger and bigger servings, and technology—automobiles, remote controls, escalators, and computers—has made it possible to entirely avoid exercise.

Twenty years ago, parents would send their children outside after school, where they'd play catch, baseball, hopscotch, and hide-and-go-seek until dinnertime. Today, they're inside playing video games or watching TV.

Calorically speaking, the difference is significant. A child who spends an hour watching television will burn 60 calories; a child playing outside (team sports, riding a bike) for an hour burns over 200. And kids watching TV, most notably in the after-school hours, are exposed to a multitude of food commercials that seduce them to snack.

Overeating junk food and inactivity make a diabolical duo that literally poisons our children's ability to handle all the excess fat and sugar they eat. Adult-onset (Type II) diabetes, a disease in which the body gradually becomes insensitive to its own insulin (the hormone cells needed to convert sugar into energy), used to strike most adults past the age of forty-five. Today, 25 percent of all new cases of adult-onset diabetes are occurring in people under the age of twenty. Diabetes is the leading cause of blindness, kidney failure, and amputations. Sixteen million Americans now suffer from the disease, which kills 180,000 a year, and at least a third of those with type II diabetes are unaware they have the illness.

Dr. Gerald Bernstein, president of the American Diabetes Association, comments: "What we are learning, unfortunately, is this is now a disease of children. Type 2 diabetes is making alarming gains among youth because of rising childhood obesity and the prevalence of sedentary lifestyles." Diabetes already costs about $100 billion annually, more than heart disease, cancer, or AIDS.

Children tend to think themselves invulnerable, and they can't see the long-term risks of their eating behavior and lack of exercise. Parents are lulled into this same false sense of security when it comes to their children; after all, how many kids have heart attacks? But we can no longer delay dealing with these problems.

EXERCISE ALONE IS NOT ENOUGH

It's a Friday at 8:30 A.M. and Ean Meyer, head coach in charge of player development at the Evert Tennis Academy in Boca Raton, Florida, is looking at a twelve-hour day and a court full of eager students. Ean, who looks like a South African version of Crocodile Dundee, is also the academy's unofficial pied piper–meets–Marine Corps drill sergeant. His students—not just ordinary kids, mind you, but tomorrow's tennis champions—execute his every command in lockstep as he begins the day's training with a Simon says–type drill, the tennis equivalent of synchronized swimming. "Up-down-up, up-down-up," echoes across the court as Ean's charges raise and lower their racquets in hypnotic, if not reverential, compliance.

"Ean is incredible with kids," confides Chris Evert, the academy's tennis legend-in-residence. "He's the best."

There are hundreds of well-heeled parents who are literally banking on Chris's judgment. Having paid upward of $25,000 a year to put their child through her demanding-but-chic tennis boot camp, they expect their investment to pay off. Most are highly motivated, focused-on-success parents; many can already envision their little darling brandishing the winner's cup at center court, Wimbledon, while thanking Mom and Dad for making it all possible.

•

It's now Friday at 8:30 P.M., and Ean Meyer has logged another twelve-hour day. The Evert Academy is empty, peaceful, and dark, save for a single lighted court where Ean gathers up his equipment. He has just put me through one of his infamous drill-till-you-drop workouts.

"You know, some of these overanxious parents need to be coached, just like their kids," Ean quips half jokingly. "Many of them tend to live vicariously through their children. They want their kid to be a success, but they shouldn't let parental pressure ruin the fun. Children will rebel and drop out of sports. These kids have enough to worry about without the Pressure Monster rearing its ugly head."

"But that's not the main problem," he continues. "I see many of these kids getting tired every day after lunch. They tend to lose their concentration on the court and their learning suffers. Some are even getting fatter, despite all the training and tennis they play each day," he complains. "We have an exercise physiologist, physiotherapist, sports psychologist, and some of the world's best coaches in residence, but we are clearly missing a vital piece of the fitness puzzle."

"Yes," I tell him. "The most important piece—the Ultimate Ratio."

DIABETES INCREASE LINKED TO TEEN FATNESS

Ten years ago, few people under the age of forty were even screened for diabetes, which is why health researchers named the disease adult-onset diabetes. Literally overnight, an increasing number of happy-go-lucky teens are being diagnosed with adult-onset (Type II) diabetes. In a regional medical center where I used to counsel patients, four out of five new cases of Type II diabetics were children.

Health experts note that minority children are particularly at risk. Parents of overfat black, Hispanic, and American Indian children should particularly be on the lookout for diabetes symptoms. Pediatricians must also screen for this disease more aggressively. These medical specialists are not usually looking for diabetes in children because they weren't trained to do so.

Eating according to the Ultimate Ratio will help kids and teens normalize their body weight and thereby reduce the risk of getting this "adult" disease at an early age. I predict that one day all school lunch programs will be structured according to the nutritional principles of the Ultimate Ratio. But you can start today to reduce the risk that your children will get this debilitating disease by teaching them to eat according to the Ultimate Ratio.

BLOOD PRESSURE RISING IN KIDS AND TEENS

In addition to increasing body size and body fat, blood pressure is rising among U.S. adolescents between the ages of ten and fourteen. This means today's kids will be tomorrow's heart attack and stroke victims. If we do not pay attention to these trends, we may well see an increase in cardiovascular morbidity and mortality rates as the children become adults.

This trend among our kids and teens is the result of large increases in average body weight accompanied by relatively small changes in height, and it affects all races and both genders, with the exception of Hispanic girls.

The increases in systolic blood pressure may be directly caused, at least in part, by increased weight. High blood pressure often originates in youth. You may recall that I failed my military physical examination because of high blood pressure. Increases in blood pressure during adolescence are an important predictor of subsequent adult hypertension.

PARENTS: ROLE MODELS OR OBESITY MODELS?

Do you know what the most important predictor of childhood obesity is? It's fat parents.

Are you fat? There's a pretty good chance you are: The vast majority of American adults are above their ideal weight, and over a third of them are clinically obese. You are the role model for fitness and health your child will look to first. You don't have to be in perfect shape, but you should practice what you preach with respect to food choices and activity levels.

Obesity actually begins in the cradle. Sadly, many American mothers have misconceptions about feeding their infants that increase the chances their children will become obese. A recent study by Johns Hopkins researchers revealed that many mothers, especially those from lower-income families, believe a heavier infant is a healthier one (healthy breast-fed two-year-olds tend to be a little chunky, but that is a temporary condition). Some introduced cereal and other solid foods as early as one month because they thought milk alone would not satisfy their child's hunger. And as their children got older, most of the mothers in the study continued to soothe them with food—feeding them in response to difficult behaviors unassociated with hunger (e.g., fussiness, irritability, and crying).

Many health experts believe that after age five, the situation really boils down to this: Kids and teens eat too much and exercise too little. In thermodynamic terms, they take in more calories than they burn, and store the excess as fat.

But is it really as simple as that?

Actually, it's a more complex story, one that reveals an inherent conflict of interest between a lucrative weight-loss industry and an even bigger and more aggressive packaged-food industry. It is the battle of thousands of spas across the nation full of exercise machines against a burgeoning technology of labor-saving devices. It's a war for our children's free time: Surfing the Internet is the sport of choice of many teens, supplanting baseball, soccer, basketball, and other sports as the primary after-school activity. Finally, it's the inborn preference for fat and sugar constantly stimulated by an endless barrage of junk food advertisements and unhealthy school lunch menus.

Science and technology have made it easy for kids and teens to grow fat (many of today's kids have never even manually opened a car window), but we can't lay all of the blame for our kids' fatness and lack of fitness on society. Kids first learn eating habits from their parents. This places the burden of keeping kids fit squarely on the shoulders of parents. And although we all want our children to be fit, recent studies indicate that while more adults are at the health clubs, their children are sitting at home.

Dining outside the home creates more problems. We take our kids out to dinner and order such dishes as fettuccine Alfredo, which the Center for Science in the Public Interest calls "a heart attack on a plate." At the movie theater, we treat them to tubs of oil-soaked movie-theater popcorn, which pack a week's worth of fat into a container nearly as big as a fire bucket, or buy them Godzilla-size candy bars to snack on as they *sit* watching the movie. Then we bring home pints of super-fatted Ben & Jerry's ice cream and snack on Mrs. Field's chocolate chip cookies, two of which contain the artery-clogging equivalent of half a stick of butter.

Most kids eat until they clean their plates—behavior they learn from their parents at the dining room table and when dining out. Given the size of restaurant servings these days, that is an increasingly dangerous habit. As fast-food giants and theme restaurants have cultivated peoples' tastes for behemoth-sized burgers and sumptuous shakes, America has turned into one big gulp.

Too often, we eat out of emotional needs, not just hunger, and we teach our children to do the same. We eat when we're happy; we eat when we're sad. Most of us use food as a substitute for many other things. Food is our ever-present friend. It's a soothing source of solace and satisfaction. We teach our kids to use food in the same ways.

Even athletic parents who serve as excellent role models for a healthy lifestyle can't control their childrens' diets 100 percent of the time. How can parental advice for moderation compete against commercial offerings like BigFoot pizzas, Burger King Whoppers, and Wendy's Biggie Fries?

The bad news is: It can't. The good news is: It doesn't always have to.

LET THEM EAT CAKE

Your kids are in bed, and you finally have time to clean up the kitchen. Cluttering the counter are the remains of the day's snacks—empty cans of soda, half-eaten cookies, and candy bar wrappers. "That's it," you say to yourself. "Tomorrow, no more junk food, no more snacks!"

In reality, however, a no-junk food/no-snacks policy is unrealistic and self-defeating. Snacking is a major part of the adolescent lifestyle, and may provide on average 20 percent of a teen's daily calories. With the Ultimate Ratio recipes, you can make snacks and fast meals that look and taste like the nutritionally naughty foods kids crave: hamburgers, hot dogs, chicken nuggets, and milk shakes. These healthy snacks and meals are based on a new generation of functional foods that look and taste like the real thing. They contain only good stuff, such as cancer-fighting phytonutrients, muscle-building protein, heart-healthy fiber, and peak-performance vitamins and minerals.

In a perfect world, food manufacturers would cease making soft drinks, doughnuts, candy, and ice cream; Chinese restaurants would cook with no oil, Italian restaurants would dish up fat-free tomato sauce, and McDonald's would replace their Big Macs with McSoy Macs. Your kids would all eat perfectly, exercise regularly, and stay at their perfect weight. There's just one hitch to achieving this nutritional Nirvana:

Kids will be kids.

This simple and universal truth means that you can nag, cajole, threaten, harass, and demand until your face turns blue, but your kids will almost always wind up eating some junk. That's just a fact of life. You don't eat perfectly, and your kids won't either.

You'll get better results, in most cases, by making measured improvements in your child's diet rather than by trying to completely reform it. Instead of cutting out the traditional fatty "forbiddens" altogether, you can balance them with the healthy snacks and meals based on the soy foods and functional foods forming the backbone of the Ultimate Ratio eating strategy. Instead of eliminating snacks and junk food, the Ultimate Ratio lets you plan them—in a new and healthy way.

NO SOY FOR CHILDREN WITH ASTHMA AND/OR AN ALLERGY TO PEANUTS

Soy, like its cousin the peanut, has been linked in a small number of severe and potentially fatal cases of food allergy, particularly in children with asthma who are also very sensitive to peanuts. A recent Swedish study has uncovered a possible link between soy consumption and food allergies. The study's authors concluded that soy "has probably been underestimated as a cause of food anaphylaxis" and suggest that food labels clearly state when foods contain soy protein.

Between 1993 and 1996, four deaths in Sweden were attributed to soy, say the researchers. All four of the children who died from soy anaphylaxis were allergic to peanuts but had no known allergy to soy.

It appears that children most at risk for developing a severe reaction to soy products already have asthma and a severe allergy to peanuts, say the researchers. In cases where the allergy was fatal, the amount of soy consumed varied between 1 and 10 grams—an amount commonly found in commercially prepared meats and soy meat replacers and soy beverages. "Such an amount may occur in hidden form in ordinary hamburgers, meatballs, kebabs, sausages, and bread, but rarely in other foods," note the researchers. They concluded: "It seems reasonable to advise persons at risk to avoid foods known to contain soy, and to avoid hamburgers, meatballs, and similar food if they cannot be guaranteed free from soy. Peanuts should not be served in schools and nursery schools, and the labeling of foods containing soy protein should be improved."

PARENTS AS SOLE AGENTS OF DIET CHANGE FOR THEIR CHILDREN

The family meal table should serve as much more than a mere filling station; you can use it to establish the ground rules for eating to win. Child development experts and physicians have long realized that kids whose families regularly gather for meals are in better overall health (and make better students) than those from families eating catch-as-catch-can style.

When it comes to weight control, parents often assume that what's good for an adult is good for a child, but doctors and child-care experts rarely recommend that an overweight child lose weight: Placing a child on a weight-loss diet can interfere with growth, lead to self-image problems, and produce such eating disorders as anorexia nervosa and bulimia, especially in girls. Instead, health professionals like to see children and teens grow into their weight by making smarter food choices and getting plenty of exercise.

A family-based approach to diet and exercise—one where the parents are the primary agents of change rather than the children—increases the likelihood of success. Recent studies have shown that a family-based approach is far superior to a child-based diet: The dropout rate in family-based therapy is nine times lower and the amount of weight lost is almost twice as great compared to therapy programs where the child is the sole agent of change.

The family-based approach, in which the parents are the sole agent of change, has several advantages over conventional diet programs, in which children are the sole agent of change:

- A higher compliance (lower dropout) rate;
- Increased weight loss;
- Better maintenance of weight loss;
- Potential weight loss in parents;
- Cost effectiveness;
- Avoidance of psychological problems associated with conventional weight loss treatments for children.

The reasons for this remarkable difference can be explained by the lower level of resistance to change by children because the weight loss–related decisions were not theirs. In a family-based approach the child is not treated as a patient; the family is treated as a whole. It is parents who assume the responsibility for reducing the entire family's exposure to food stimuli, introducing functional foods to replace unhealthy foods, and creating opportunities for physical exercise. Through their active participation, obese parents may also lose weight.

Parents of children under two years old shouldn't even think about altering their infants' or toddlers' diet (children under two should be given full-fat soy milk or whole milk after being weaned from breast milk or formula, because of their higher need for dietary fat). Even if an infant or toddler seems heavier than normal, cutting back on feedings isn't recommended, unless done under medical supervision. Children of this age are going through significant developmental changes; they need sufficient calories, vitamins, minerals, and fats. Calorie deprivation could impair growth.

For overweight children from the age of two and up, there are simple dietary changes that parents can make:

- Substitute soy meat replacement foods for red meats;
- Replace snack chips with low-sodium pretzels;
- Serve soda only on special occasions;
- Keep a bowl of fresh fruit available, and cut it up for the kids;
- Substitute skim milk or non-fat soy milk for whole milk;
- Reduce juice consumption. Juice can significantly contribute to childhood weight gain (recall that eating too much sugar can turn off fat burning). A recent study published in *Pediatrics,* the journal of the American Academy of Pediatrics, found that preschoolers who drank a cup and a half of juice or more per day were twice as likely to be overweight as those who drank less. Many kids easily consume between 500 to 1,000 extra calories a day in juice. That's significant, considering that children who consume 300 calories worth of juice more than they burn off every day will gain five extra pounds in a year. Children who continue to gain weight at that rate could, by age ten, be 50 percent above their ideal weight.

ENCOURAGING PHYSICAL ACTIVITY IN CHILDREN

Physical activity and sports, along with diet, form the foundation of a healthy lifestyle for children no matter what their age. As a parent, you can help your child develop the skills and interest in sports that contribute to lifelong fitness. You should also strive to set a good example by participating in your own fitness program, teaching your child the skills you know, and encouraging him or her to develop additional skills and seek professional coaching if he or she shows talent for a particular sport.

AGES 3 TO 5

During this period, children develop their basic movement skills. This is a critical time for developing a foundation that will help your child succeed in sports and fitness throughout life. Emphasize movement in your child's play, incorporating such skills as tossing and catching a ball, hitting a ball with a bat or tennis racquet, jumping, and running.

AGES 5 TO 8

Children in this age group develop basic motor skills to build more complex movements. This is a perfect time to teach them bicycling, skating, and swimming. Get your child involved in organized group or team play, which will help build self-confidence and learn the value of teamwork. Children should be exposed to a variety of sports and physical activities in order to let them decide which ones they enjoy the most.

AGES 8 TO 12

This is a critical time for children to sustain a high level of physical activity. During these ages, children tend to become inactive, especially if they like computer games. Children eight to twelve are greatly influenced by their peers, who often determine which physical activities and sports they will embrace. These can also be awkward years. Children at this age generally lack the anabolic hormones required to develop large muscles, but regular physical activity can strengthen their cardiovascular system, muscles, and bones. If your children show little interest in sports, encourage them to engage in such individual activities as biking, hiking, swimming, and rollerblading.

AGES 13 TO 18

Once puberty kicks in, many children may become competitive and even dream of becoming professional athletes. This competitiveness simply reflects a healthy attitude toward physical fitness, and you should encourage your child's interest and help him/her find the appropriate level at which to play or compete. Lessons from a professional can help children develop the sports skills that will help them enjoy exercise for the rest of their lives. Inactivity during the teen years can predispose kids to a lifelong sedentary lifestyle. If you are not physically active, now is the time to set an example and get involved in a sport or join a family-oriented gym. As a beginning, try to plan family walks whenever possible.

CAFFEINE AND KIDS

Caffeine and related compounds are found in many brands of soft drinks, bottled teas, coffee, tea, cocoa, chocolate, and even aspirin compounds. Caffeine has been shown to improve alertness, hand-eye coordination, and performance of various tasks. But what amount of caffeine, if any, is safe for kids and teens?

Almost all caffeine studies conclude that moderate use (the equivalent of up to 4 cups of coffee per day) poses no serious risks, such as cancer, heart disease, or diabetes to most healthy adults (notwithstanding caffeine allergies or sensitivity). But caffeine has not been as thoroughly tested with children. The potency of caffeine, like any other drug, depends on body weight, and since kids weigh less than adults, the effects of the drug can be more pronounced. Studies have shown that consumption of caffeinated beverages can leach the calcium from bones in adults. If children consume such beverages, the calciuric losses can be significant, especially if the drink contains sugar. For example, when investigators gave a test group of 13- to 18-year-olds an unsweetened caffeinated drink, their urinary calcium output increased by 25 percent. When they drank caffeine plus sugar, their calcium loss rose even more. Phosphorus and sugar, found in most colas, accelerate bone loss even more.

Drinking just one can of a caffeinated soft drink can cause a child to lose as much as 120 milligrams of calcium (most health experts recommend 1,200 milligrams/day for growing kids). Furthermore, a soft drink after a workout can deplete sodium, chloride, and potassium from muscle cells, which could increase muscle soreness and delay recovery time after exercise. Caffeine is okay when used occasionally (such as in hot cocoa, milk chocolate, tea, and smart drinks like the **Orange Genius** on page 166), but daily caffeine intake should be restricted to no more than 50 milligrams, and no more than two to three times per week. Those who want to be sure of obtaining adequate calcium can take a multivitamin and mineral supplement, which contains at least 250 milligrams calcium and 100 milligrams magnesium. This will more than offset daily calcium losses due to nutritional factors that promote calcium excretion, such as caffeinated beverages and high-sodium foods. Encourage your children to drink any sweetened beverages through a straw. That will help preserve their tooth enamel and reduce the risk of dental caries.

CHOCOLATE IS OKAY FOR MOST KIDS

The Ultimate Ratio allows you to eat a small amount of milk chocolate as a treat. But chocolate contains caffeine and related compounds. So is milk chocolate really safe for kids? Here are some popular myths and truths about chocolate:

Chocolate makes kids hyperactive: Myth. Parents worry that if their kids eat chocolate they'll start zipping around the house. While there are caffeinelike compounds in chocolate, they won't make kids hyperactive unless they eat too much of it. One ounce of milk chocolate has as much caffeine as a cup of decaffeinated coffee. The sugar content of chocolate is more likely to keep kids energized than the caffeine. It's okay to allow your kids to eat small amounts of the sweet stuff when you limit intake to such special occasions as birthdays, Halloween, and a movie outing.

It causes acne: Myth. Consuming chocolate does not cause pimples or acne. Scientific studies show that there's no relationship between chocolate and acne. Acne during the teen years is brought on by hormonal fluctuation.

It causes weight gain: Myth. Some parents worry about their children gaining weight during holidays such as Halloween. Munching on a little extra candy once in a while won't make a child overweight as long as parents limit snacks once the Halloween bounty is gone.

It causes tooth decay: Yes and No. The sugar in candy can cause cavities, but research has shown that compounds in chocolate can discourage the growth of cavity-causing bacteria. To minimize the problem, children should brush their teeth soon after eating candy. The longer that sugar stays on the teeth, the more damage it can do. Avoiding chewy caramels and toffees will help, since they may be harder to remove with brushing.

It raises blood levels of cholesterol: Myth. A number of dietitians I've spoken to believe that the fats in milk chocolate raise cholesterol levels in the blood. This is not true, as established by recent research showing that the addition of a chocolate candy bar to the Step I diet designed by the American Heart Association to lower cholesterol did not raise cholesterol levels. In fact, the addition of the chocolate bar actually raised beneficial HDL-cholesterol levels.

A lifetime of enjoying chocolate may help us live longer. Harvard School of Public Health researchers have discovered that men who ate chocolate regularly from about the age of sixty-five lived nearly a year longer than those who avoided sweets. Death rates were lowest among those eating chocolate and other sweets one to three times a month, but highest among those who abstained. The researchers studied the men for five years. Even after researchers took into account other factors such as smoking, the results were the same. This study looked only at the effects of eating chocolate in older men. There is reason to believe that a lifelong habit of enjoying the seductive sweet candy might yield even more impressive results.

How does eating chocolate extend life? One answer can be found in the phytonutrients, called phenols, in chocolate. Phenols are powerful antioxidants that deactivate harmful free radicals linked to disease and aging. A 1.5-ounce chunk of milk chocolate contains the same antioxidant dose as a heart-friendly 5-ounce glass of red wine.

If chocolate is indeed responsible for this longevity effect, there may be yet another explanation: Eating it simply makes people feel good. Neuropharmacologists have shown that eating chocolate releases cannabinoids in the brain—compounds similar to those responsible for the high induced by smoking marijuana.

An occasional bite of chocolate or cup of cocoa is okay for most kids. As long as you limit consumption to about once a week, chocolate and cocoa can help sweeten the disposition of just about any child who loves the taste.

6

MUSCLE CANDY AND
PERFORMANCE NUTRIENTS

Baron Pierre de Coubertin, the Frenchman who revived the Olympic games of ancient Greece, never heard of the sports nutrition supplement, creatine monohydrate. In his day, most athletes took a more primitive approach to competition—they simply played to win. When the Baron chose as a motto for the modern Olympics *"Citius, altius, fortius"*—"Swifter, higher, stronger"—he couldn't possibly have imagined that the ability to achieve the Olympic credo would come from a bottle.

In a world where the difference between winning and losing is measured in hundredths or even thousandths of a second, athletes now swallow just about anything that promises to give them a competitive edge—including large doses of hype surrounding the latest headline-grabbing sports performance boosters. Most performance enhancers turn out to be ineffective. In the worst cases, as with anabolic steroids and amphetamines, they may pack more poison than punch.

Do any of today's power potions really make a difference in strength, endurance, and performance? If so, which ones can you use to safely and effectively build better muscles? Which ones will actually make you run faster, jump higher, and go farther?

First, I'll tell you about the safe and effective all-natural performance enhancers that I've used with great success to help athletes. Then I'll show you how to put them all together to create your own peak performance program—one that will give you the edge in competition—on the court, at the office, or in the classroom. But first, we must ask ourselves an important question . . .

ARE SPORTS SUPPLEMENTS FAIR?

Critics of the energy-from-a-bottle mentality argue that using anything other than ordinary food and water to boost sports performance corrupts the purity of competition. If that's true, then athletic nobility has been sullied for thousands of years, because the champions of the original Olympiad were not above swigging a concoction made from deer liver extract in an attempt to run more swiftly than their competition.

Today, exercise physiologists, coaches, and trainers employ the latest scientific knowledge to help athletes develop advanced training techniques and maximum fitness for each of the twenty-nine sports in the Olympic Games. Biomechanical experts use computers attached to high-tech cameras and sensors to study the dynamics of movement. Design engineers employ sophisticated materials to create streamlined racing bicycles and powerful, almost lighter-than-air tennis racquets. Sports psychologists teach athletes how to think to win with Zenlike mental-training techniques. Why should sports nutrition be held to a loftier standard? If a substance made by the body itself can take an athlete higher, faster, and farther, is it really unfair to encapsulate it, wash it down with a glass of Gatorade (a performance-enhancing sports drink), and head off for the next track meet or triathlon?

I believe that any *nonhormonal* nutrient or chemical compound made by the human body or any compound found in natural foods that studies have shown to be safe and effective should be considered fair and legal by all major governing sports bodies.* If athletes can use synthetic, high-tech sports equipment to improve their performance, then, surely, they should be allowed to consume a natural substance manufactured by their own bodies. After all, metal alloys and other performance-boosting polymers came into existence only recently, but the body's own ergogenic compounds have been with us since the beginning of humankind.

---

*Hormones are powerful, druglike compounds that can be dangerous when used in even small amounts and therefore should be banned from use in athletic competition. Unless you have been advised to take them by a physician for a medical reason, avoid these substances. Hormones make bad medicine for healthy athletes.

It's not the body's natural performance enhancers that pose the biggest threat to fairness in competition and wellness in athletes. The real problem arises when profit-hungry sports supplement companies attempt to capitalize on the feeding frenzy that follows the newest flavor-of-the-month supplement before science has had a chance to catch up with hype. The national media fan the flames of controversy, creating the kind of headlines that help popularize unproven supplements. The challenge is for athletes to maintain restraint until researchers have determined the safety and efficacy of the claims made by manufacturers and users of these supplements. As you will learn, only a small number of performance-enhancing supplements pass the acid test of scientific scrutiny.

CREATINE POWER: MYTH OR MUSCLE MAGIC?

Most people consume about 1 to 2 grams of creatine a day, primarily from meat and seafood. But the amount required to boost muscular strength far exceeds what we can get from diet alone. Eastern bloc Olympic athletes, aware of this dietary shortcoming, started gulping the tasteless white powder during the early 1980s in an effort to bulk up and beat the competition.

Creatine users usually experience dramatic weight gains—not as unsightly fat but rather as extra water. Most studies have found that an initial loading dose of 20 grams followed by 2 to 5 grams a day can lead to packing on as much as 20 to 30 pounds within a few months. No amount of creatine, however, will bulge the biceps of a sedentary slug—you still have to work out to bulk up.

While a number of studies on creatine supplementation demonstrate that brief supplementation improves anaerobic athletic performance (e.g., those activities requiring short bursts of power), it is not at all clear that continuing supplementation produces any further benefits. So there is, as yet, no justification for taking creatine on an ongoing basis. The risks and benefits of taking creatine supplements indefinitely remain unknown.

Creatine isn't for all athletes. It probably won't help distance runners because of the large weight gain it causes, and it's not a good idea for anyone trying to maximize their power-to-weight ratio. I suspect many runners don't relish the idea of carrying twenty extra pounds up Heartbreak Hill in the next Boston Marathon. Cyclists would also face the same power-to-weight ratio problem, as would swimmers, since weight gain could adversely affect body position in the water.

The news on creatine isn't beefy enough to garner the unqualified blessing of all sports physicians, trainers, and national health organizations. Few fitness experts are prepared to go out on a limb and sing the praises of creatine, because if and when the bough breaks—and that could eventually happen with more comprehensive scientific scrutiny—they aren't willing to take the fall. Still, there's money to be made, both by the supplement companies that sell the stuff and the athletes who are betting their health that a creatine milkshake a day can keep fatigue away. After all, Mark McGwire, the 250-pound poster boy for creatine, used the white powder to help him set a world record in 1998 for most home runs in a single season. Sadly, McGwire also used a steroidal hormone called androstenedione, an over-the-counter compound that can lead to serious hormonal imbalance in the body; creatine is not a hormone, but an ordinary amino acid–like compound found in foods. By doing so, he tarnished an otherwise spectacular achievement. "Andro," as it's called on the street, is banned by the International Olympic Committee and a growing list of national sports organizations; hopefully, it will soon be proscribed by all governing sports bodies. McGwire was lucky, and so his record will stand—but with a footnote to indicate that he slugged his way into the record books with hormonal help.

MINDING YOUR Ps AND Qs

Creatine could turn out be the spinach of the new century, but nearly two decades before Mark McGwire launched the home run heard 'round the world—and the creatine controversy—Eastern European bloc Olympic athletes were gleefully gulping down this muscle candy like kids in a candy store. And, like McGwire, the Olympic competitors mixed their creatine with more powerful and dangerous steroid compounds.

So what's the big deal over creatine? Why do casual and professional athletes sing its praises in the press and plunk down collectively more than $100 million a year to get a taste of the tasteless white powder? Understanding the science and appeal behind creatine's muscle magic, it turns out, is simply a question of minding one's Ps and Qs.

ATP: Adenosine Triphosphate

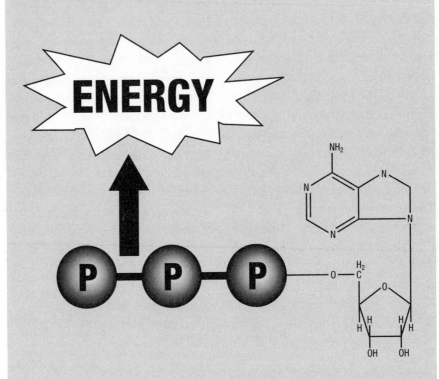

Remember when I told you how plants capture the energy of the sun and store it in carbo-hydrates? Here's where that usable energy ultimately winds up—in ATP. The terminal phosphate (P) bond of ATP, which binds the second and third phosphate groups, eagerly awaits its fifteen nanoseconds of fame. When the call for energy comes, enzymes split the terminal P from ATP, releasing the solar energy stored in that bond so that you can run, jump, think, and read this sentence.

FIRST, THE Ps

You've already learned how important carbohydrates are to peak athletic per-formance, but now you're going learn just how important ATP can be to any-one who aspires to fitness and optimal health.

All living cells, from those found in the lowliest bacteria up to our own, contain ATP (adenosine triphosphate), the mother of all energy compounds. Cells that require maximum energy, including those in the brain, heart, and muscle tissues, contain the highest amounts of ATP.

ATP spells energy for an athlete. But too little of the compound spells disaster for endurance athletes and those engaged in lengthy competition: the harder and heavier you exercise, the quicker you use up your supply of ATP.

It's the "P" in ATP that is the business end of the molecule. There are actually three "Ps" (phosphate atoms) in ATP, but it's the energy stored in the chemical bond of the terminal P that puts the punch in this power molecule. The muscle magic begins when ATP surrenders its terminal P, releasing the energy that drives muscular contraction.

If you can keep regenerating ATP at the rate your exercising muscles use it up, you will dramatically delay the onset of fatigue and outlast your competition. ATP is an energy molecule designed to take you the distance—a very long distance, if you can make enough of it. But once ATP levels drop by about 30 percent, muscles fatigue and power output diminishes.

There's another energy compound like ATP, called CP (creatine phosphate), made by the body in small amounts and stored in muscle cells. During high-intensity exercise, energy for reconstituting ATP is met by the concomitant breakdown of CP and the energy derived from burning carbohydrates (yet another reason for shunning a high-protein/low-carb diet). So the real value of creatine supplementation is to increase the amount of CP stored in muscle tissue, which, in a trained athlete, is usually about three to four times that of ATP. Since a 400-meter race will use up 90 percent of the body's CP reserves, supplementary creatine and supporting nutrients could be helpful for athletic competition that lasts beyond several minutes. I say could, because no one is absolutely certain at this point.

BOOSTING CREATINE'S EFFECTIVENESS

You've learned how ATP and CP can power your muscles by releasing energy in the terminal P-group chemical bond. You've learned that by taking supplementary creatine, you can increase the amount of CP in muscles beyond what is possible with ordinary foods. But there is one more trick that you can use—one that Mark McGwire didn't know about—to achieve the maximum amount of CP storage in muscles.

You don't have to be a biochemist to see that the difference between creatine and creatine phosphate is, well, phosphate! So if you decide to supplement with creatine, might it be a good idea to supplement with phosphate as well?

The answer is maybe. I've been using a phosphate drink called Quick-Fix (Endurance brand, which can be ordered through most General Nutrition Centers and natural food markets) phosphate salts for the last fourteen years to help world-class athletes eat to win. Study results on phosphate loading are mixed. Some find that it boosts endurance; others find no effect at all. Phosphate salts have been used by the military as far back as World War I to give fatigued footsoldiers an energy boost. Even though the jury is still out on phosphate salts, if you supplement with creatine you might want to use

HMB: Creatine's Bridesmaid

Okay, so maybe you're not quite ready to split a creatine milkshake with Mark McGwire. You don't have to if you know about HMB. If you want to build muscle (or at least stop losing the muscle you already have) and burn fat, HMB may be an effective way to bulk up and slim down. You may not have heard of HMB (short for beta-hydroxy-beta-methyl-butyrate) because the media hasn't given it nearly the ink it has given to creatine.

HMB is found in muscle cells (it's a metabolite of the amino acid L-leucine) and helps prevent the breakdown of muscle. Some of the first studies on HMB conducted at Vanderbilt University and at Iowa State University found that HMB increased strength and lean body mass in athletes. Since both universities hold patents on HMB and have licensed its production and distribution to dietary supplement manufacturers, the findings of these early studies must be looked at with a degree of skepticism.

HMB is classified as a dietary supplement because it occurs naturally in such diverse foods as catfish and citrus fruits. HMB plays a role in muscle building and fat burning, but only in response to exercise. A recent study by researchers at State University of New York at Stony Brook revealed that when muscle cells were exposed to HMB in a test tube, they burned fat faster. This study, together with a growing body of research, suggests that athletes may be able to use HMB to build muscle and burn fat more efficiently for fuel, decrease stored body fat, and spare protein and carbohydrate for muscle building and energy production, respectively. More research is needed, however, to confirm the long-term safety and efficacy of this natural compound.

Some researchers believe that HMB regulates enzymes responsible for muscle-tissue breakdown. This theory is supported by evidence that HMB supplementation decreased biochemical indicators of muscle breakdown among weight lifters. Check with a physician before using this or any other dietary supplement.

them as well. In a recent study at Old Dominion University, six trained male cyclists and triathletes ingested either one gram of sodium phosphate or a glucose placebo four times daily for three days prior to a maximal cycling test. The phosphate-supplemented athletes experienced a significant increase in endurance performance in all tests when compared to those who did the same tests without phosphate loading.

Will phosphate salts work for you? Tennis champion Andre Agassi believes they work for him. Eat-to-Winners have been using *Quick-Fix* for the last fourteen years to boost their endurance and fight fatigue. Isn't it time you tried one of these performance-enhancing supplements or drinks?

AND NOW, THE Qs

After learning about the three most important Ps—ATP, CP, and phosphate—we also need to mind our Qs. In this case, Q stands for coenzyme Q_{10}, a nutrient that helps transfer energy to ATP in cells.

No one had ever heard of coenzyme Q_{10} (CoQ_{10}) until 1956, when scientists at the University of Wisconsin discovered it lurking in beef heart mitochondria (mitochondria are membrane-bound structures within cells, where fat, protein, and carbohydrate can be converted into energy, then stored in ATP). Since that time, scientists have detected abnormally low levels of CoQ_{10} levels in people who suffer from a wide variety of ailments, including heart disease, muscular dystrophy, and cancer. CoQ_{10} serves three major functions: It helps transfer energy derived from the breakdown of foods to ATP; it quenches free radicals generated in the energy-making process; and it helps protect the integrity of the mitochondrial membrane.

The last time you enjoyed a tuna fish sandwich, you got a small dose of CoQ_{10}. It takes six vitamins and trace minerals to make CoQ_{10} in the body and, like creatine, you'd have to eat about 16 pounds of beef to obtain a peak performance dose. Competitive athletes take between 30 and 120 milligrams a day to saturate their muscle tissue with the compound. CoQ_{10} is found in beef, mackerel, peanuts, salmon, sardines, spinach, and tuna. You might think that vegetarians would be at risk of a CoQ_{10} deficiency, but such is not the case. Vegetarians typically have more than double the level of CoQ_{10} in their blood plasma than omnivores, so it seems that a diet high in vegetables and fruits promotes CoQ_{10} preservation.

CoQ_{10} itself is not an ergogenic compound, and taking it alone won't help you run faster or farther. It works in conjunction with a number of other energy compounds to create ATP:

L-Carnitine: You simply can't burn fat unless you have enough L-carnitine in your cells. L-carnitine helps transport fatty acids through the cell membrane into the mitochondria within the cell, where they are burned to produce cellular energy that can be used to make ATP. By promoting the burning of fat, L-carnitine spares proteins and carbohydrates from being catabolized and used as muscular fuels. Hence, L-carnitine spares the breakdown of muscle tissue. Although your body can manufacture a certain amount of L-carnitine each day, research has shown that certain conditions, such as aging, exercise, stress, illness, and alcohol ingestion, can deplete your body's supply of L-carnitine. Studies have shown that endurance athletes given L-carnitine (2 grams orally twice each day) during a four-week period of training showed a significant increase in the activities of energy enzymes responsible for synthesizing ATP. When the athletes were given a placebo, no significant changes in enzyme levels were observed. Acetyl-L-carnitine, a closely related compound, is more effectively absorbed into the bloodstream and cells than regular L-carnitine.* Athletes generally take 1 to 3 grams of L-carnitine each day. L-carnitine should be taken on an empty stomach for maximum absorption. Acetyl-L-carnitine increases the ability of brain cells to utilize alternative energy sources when normal glucose update is impaired, such as in the later stages of endurance competition. Animal flesh has the highest carnitine content, especially steak and ground beef. Vegetables, fruits, and grains provide relatively small amounts of carnitine, so people who don't eat red meats may want to take carnitine supplements.

L-Carnosine: The fact that L-carnosine is highly concentrated in muscle tissue indicates its important role in controlling muscle contractions. Even though carnosine isn't directly involved in the synthesis of ATP, it is intimately involved in increasing the concentration of enzymes that allow ATP to release its energy. The complete biological role of carnosine remains to be

---

*Acetyl-L-carnitine is the acetylated ester of the amino acid L-carnitine. Acetyl-L-carnitine is absorbed from the small intestine more efficiently than L-carnitine, passes more effectively through cell membranes, and is utilized more efficiently in the mitochondria of the cell.

discovered, but the list of its uses keeps growing as researchers discover new roles for the amazing nutrient, including the protection of muscle tissue and DNA from free-radical damage. Carnosine is able to prolong the lifespan potential of skin fibroblasts (cells that renew skin) and helps to revitalize skin cells that have advanced toward senescence. These functions suggest carnosine's potential use in improving wound healing and recovery from sports injuries. Dosage commonly used: 500 mg/day.

NADH: Researchers are just beginning to investigate NADH for its role in boosting athletic performance. Meat, poultry, and yeast are the most plentiful sources of NADH, although the compound occurs naturally in all plant and animal foods. Food processing, cooking, and stomach acids can destroy much of the NADH present in most foods. Like CoQ_{10}, NADH is involved in the synthesis of ATP. Supplemental NADH can boost production of the neurotransmitter dopamine, a chemical messenger vital for short-term memory, movement, muscle tone, and spontaneous physical reactions. NADH also promotes the synthesis of another neurotransmitter, norepinephrine, which contributes to alertness, concentration, and mental focus. When NADH is oxidized in mitochondria, it helps form water and energy. This energy is preserved as ATP. To keep up with the cellular demand for energy, the body continuously synthesizes NADH (a process that involves B-complex vitamins). In a recent study, researchers measured reaction times, physical performance, and performance quality in seventeen competitive cyclists and long-distance runners. The athletes took five milligrams of NADH before breakfast each morning for four weeks. After four weeks of NADH supplementation, sixteen out of the seventeen athletes experienced improved reaction times. Physical performance improved as well. Researchers hypothesized that improved reaction times may have resulted from an increase in dopamine production that led to heightened alertness and vigilance. The study concluded that stimulation of cellular ATP production by NADH may have enhanced athletic performance. Current studies and clinical trials both in the United States and abroad are exploring NADH's full potential for improved health and athletic performance. I recommend that you let further research establish the long-term safety and efficacy of this promising supplement before using it.

WHEY PROTEIN: THE LATEST MUSCLE-MIND CANDY

A growing body of scientific literature lends support to the anecdotal claims made by many athletes that whey protein supplements improve mental performance, enhance muscular development, and boost immune system function.

Whey protein is high in the branched-chain amino acids (BCAA) leucine, isoleucine, and valine. Of the twenty dietary amino acids, only nine are indispensable (meaning they cannot be synthesized in the human body). The BCAAs constitute about 40 percent of our minimum daily requirement for indispensable dietary amino acids.

Whey, with the highest biological value of any protein, is absorbed, retained, and used in the body better than other proteins. A recent pilot study found that whey protein supplements corrected the immune suppression often seen in athletes suffering from overtraining syndrome.

Whey may also exert a positive effect on bone cell growth. A recent study found that whey stimulated protein synthesis in bone cells. Studies have also shown that animals fed whey protein powder have stronger bones than those not given the supplement.

Should you use whey supplements? Most couch potatoes using the Ultimate Ratio don't need extra protein, but professional bodybuilders, endurance athletes, and very active people could possibly benefit from using whey protein to boost their protein intake during recovery from rigorous training. People on very low-calorie diets might also benefit from using whey protein supplements to obtain sufficient protein.

CORTISOL: THE DOUBLE-EDGED HORMONE

All athletes, regardless of ability or age, face the same biochemical dilemma: To compete well, they must train hard. But the body reacts to intense exercise, as it would to any stress, by secreting cortisol—a muscle-munching hormone made in the adrenal gland perched atop each kidney. Cortisol is both bane and blessing to an athlete. In order to do its primary job, which is to maintain adequate blood pressure and blood glucose levels for the brain, cortisol must break down muscle into its component amino acids. The liver is able to convert the free amino acids to glucose, which is shuttled back to the brain and the muscles for additional energy. This is one reason why low carbohydrate diets actually work against peak performance—exercising muscles must have sufficient carbohydrate at any cost, even if it means self-cannibalization.

Primary Functions of Cortisol:

- Increase the liver's synthesis of glucose from amino acids;
- Increase the liver's breakdown of glycogen (stored carbohydrate) into sugar;
- Increase muscle protein breakdown;
- Block carbohydrate from entering muscle cells;
- Maintain blood pressure by sensitizing small arteries to the action of catecholamine hormones.

NOTE: Serum cortisol exhibits diurnal variation, with its highest concentration being after waking and then declining throughout the day.

A small amount of cortisol does a body good: It helps defeat viral infections and heal damaged tissue. Such reactions are usually beneficial, but when too much cortisol dampens the immune response, it shuts down the very process that fights deadly microbes or keeps a malignant cell from progressing into an invasive tumor.

Long-distance runners and other endurance athletes have attributed the coveted "runner's high" to endorphins—opiatelike compounds made by the brain. Actually, low cortisol levels may be as responsible as any other compound for the high. Trained athletes have a more reduced cortisol response to acute exercise than do inactive individuals. Studies show that those athletes with low cortisol levels after exercise experience greater feelings of well-being in addition to less perceived exertion than untrained individuals. A number of studies have demonstrated that increased cortisol levels are associated with negative mental states, including depression and lethargy.

BOOSTING THE TESTOSTERONE-CORTISOL RATIO

Regular exercise increases testosterone production in both men and women. Unlike cortisol, testosterone builds muscles. An athlete's challenge, therefore, is to maximize the muscle-building effects of testosterone while minimizing the muscle-wasting effects of cortisol. In other words, the higher the testosterone-cortisol ratio, the better an athlete's chance for developing and maintaining muscle and sustaining peak athletic performance.

The fly in the ointment is that strenuous training, overtraining, and high-protein-low-carbohydrate diets tend to create a low, and therefore undesirable, testosterone-cortisol (T:C) ratio. Both testosterone and cortisol are hormones made through two distinctly different metabolic pathways from the mother of all steroid hormones—cholesterol. To increase the T:C ratio, some athletes take anabolic (muscle-building) steroids, chemical first cousins of testosterone. Long-term use of anabolic steroids can actually shut down the body's production of testosterone and can also cause dreadful side effects, including male infertility, heart disease, cancer, and kidney malfunction. Steroids have no place in athletic competition. They are drugs, and therefore their use constitutes abuse.

Following rigorous physical activity, a stressful event, or an injury, the adrenal glands pour cortisol into the bloodstream. The hormone makes fatty acids from adipose available for fuel to free up blood glucose for use by the brain and, indirectly, by muscles. So is there anything an athlete can do to mitigate the destructive effects of this hormone?

Yes. Eat according to the Ultimate Ratio and use the **Purple Cow** shake (page 167) after strenuous exercise to increase your T:C ratio.

ENHANCING TENNIS AND GOLF STROKES

Of the hundreds of "sports-enhancing" supplements currently on the market, only a small number have been shown to be safe and effective. One of the best for tennis players and golfers intent on improving their strokes is my Super Choline Cocktail (page 125). Martina Navratilova and Ivan Lendl used it during matches (now you know what was in those mysterious bottles from which you always saw them drinking) to improve alertness, fight fatigue, and improve their stroke production.

Researchers at a university in Belgium recently demonstrated that a carbohydrate-caffeine drink improved several measures of tennis performance. Well-trained tennis players performed three two-hour training sessions, including drills and measures of tennis performance. They were given a placebo drink, a drink containing carbohydrate, and one containing carbohydrate and caffeine. Both carbohydrate drinks but not the placebo drink resulted in better tennis performance, especially near the end of the two-hour training session. The carbohydrate-caffeine drink resulted in fewer errors during the training session, less of a decrease in running performance drills, and less deterioration in indicators of stroke skills and stroke quality. There is every reason to believe that golfers who use a carbohydrate-caffeine drink will improve their stroke performance as well.

The Belgian study used a very basic carbohydrate-caffeine drink. My Super Choline Cocktail or the premixed Choline Cocktail (Twin Laboratories: available from General Nutrition Centers and other natural foods stores nationwide) drink mix provides superior mind-body connection nutrients in addition to carbohydrate and caffeine, such as choline and ginkgo biloba. If you want to take your strokes to the limit and cut down on errors in tennis and golf, try a choline cocktail.

7

A THIRST FOR POWER

COFFEE AND OTHER ENERGY DRINKS

Montezuma may have exacted his real revenge by introducing Spanish explorers to the art of brewing caffeinated beverages. Historical records reveal that the sixteenth-century Aztec ruler brewed a type of "coffee" as a hot drink made with cacao leaves and various spices and herbs. Okay, maybe it wasn't as sophisticated as a Starbucks Frappuccino, but it must have packed a pleasing punch because Montezuma was said to have drunk up to fifty cups of the brew each day. Today, with millions of people hooked on their morning jolt of java, Montezuma's revenge remains as a lasting legacy to his fondness for power drinks.

Coffee as we know it today has actually been a favorite form of caffeine consumption since ancient times. It is mentioned in the Koran, the holy book of Islam. Coffee originated in Africa, where the beans were used as money and consumed as food, and then became popular in the Middle East during the eleventh century. The robust bean eventually found favor among the British, where coffee was introduced originally as a medicine but then became a fashionable beverage with the establishment of a large number of coffee houses between 1670 and 1730. These houses became the place to debate political and social issues of the day, which displeased British authorities enough to shut them down. Caffeine-addicted Brits revolted, forcing the government to lift its ban on the condition that coffee shops not dispense political pamphlets. When the British government placed a tax on another popular beverage, tea, American colonists threw a tea party in Boston, and coffee soon supplanted tea as *the* patriotic beverage to drink. America warmed to the beverage so hotly that it eventually became the world's leading groundskeeper, importing more than 70 percent of the planet's coffee supply.

THE SCIENCE BEHIND THE CAFFEINE BUZZ

What's the magic behind the coveted caffeine high? Why do most people feel stimulated by a good cup of coffee? Why have they throughout history risked life and limb to safeguard and hoard the beloved bean? One reason is a compound called adenosine.

Adenosine is chemically related to the universal energy molecule, adenosine triphosphate (ATP). As nerve cells (neurons) in the brain "fire," they use energy and produce adenosine in the process. Eventually, adenosine builds up outside the neuron. As a result, the excess adenosine attaches to unique adenosine receptors on neurons. Once adenosine docks with its specific receptor, the neuron slows or stops firing. Adenosine thus acts as a natural braking mechanism to keep neurons from overfiring. So how does caffeine fit it? Almost perfectly, but not quite, and that's the key to its stimulant action.

Caffeine has a similar structure to adenosine and can fit into adenosine receptors. However, like a shirt that's one size too small, the fit is imperfect and does not cause the sedating effect of adenosine. Whenever caffeine occupies the adenosine receptor site, it blocks adenosine from acting as a brake. Caffeine literally does "get on your nerves" but not as a stimulant; it simply blocks the nerve-soothing job of adenosine. Some research indicates that caffeine and related compounds (called methylxanthines) may also enhance release of the amino acids glutamate and aspartate, which are the main excitatory neurotransmitters in the brain.*

Caffeine can work only to the degree that there are excitatory neurotransmitters present; it can't boost anything in their absence. This fact explains why coffee will not counteract extreme fatigue. It's also the reason it is hard to overdose on caffeine; there is a limit to the amount of adenosine

---

*In the brain, adenosine plays a role in inducing sleep. Sleep occurs when brain energy levels drop extremely low. Since a sleeping brain is much less active than a waking one, sleep allows the organ to replenish its energy by converting adenosine to ATP. Since adenosine secretion reflects brain cell activity, rising concentrations of this chemical may help the organ gauge how much of its energy reserves (ATP) it has burned. As concentrations of adenosine near arousal centers in the brain rise (and levels of the hormone melatonin increase), we become sleepy.

How Caffeine Wakes You Up

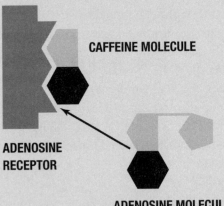

The caffeine and adenosine molecules share a common structure, as indicated by the shaded portion of the molecules.

Because of its similar shape to adenosine, the caffeine molecule can dock with the adenosine receptor on nerve cells. This action effectively blocks adenosine from connecting with its receptor and calming nerves. The docking also interferes with the ability of another calming chemical, dopamine, to bind with its receptor. Through this mechanism, caffeine literally "gets on your nerves."

Caffeine Content of Some Soft Drinks

Beverage	Mg Caffeine
Afri-Cola	100.0
Jolt	71.2
Sugar-free Mr. Pibb	58.8
Mountain Dew	55.0
Diet Mountain Dew	55.0
Kick Citrus	54
Mello Yellow	52.8
Surge	51.0
Tab	46.8
Coca-Cola	45.6
Diet Cola	45.6
Shasta Cola	44.4
Shasta Cherry Cola	44.4
Shasta Diet Cola	44.4
Mr. Pibb	40.8
OK Soda	40.5
Dr. Pepper	39.6
Pepsi Cola	37.2
Aspen	36.0
Diet Pepsi	35.4
RC Cola	36.0
Diet RC	36.0
Diet Rite	36.0
Canada Dry Cola	30.0
Canada Dry Diet Cola	1.2
7UP	0

Data from the National Soft Drink Association.

that caffeine can block. Increasing stimulatory effects with coffee occur only between one and four cups; beyond that there is little to no boost in stimulation. People who are caffeine-sensitive may feel as though they've overdosed on just half a cup of regular brewed coffee.

CAFFEINE AND FAT BURNING

Caffeine can behave as an appetite suppressant if you don't add sugar to your coffee or consume a sugary muffin or doughnut with it. It can also rev up

Caffeine Content of Coffees and Teas

Type of Coffee	Mg Caffeine
Drip	115–175
Espresso (1 serving = 1.5–2oz.)	100
Brewed	135
Instant	65–100
Decaf, brewed	3–4
Decaf, instant	2–3
Tea, iced (12 oz.)	70
Tea, brewed, imported	60
Tea, brewed, U.S.	40
Tea, instant	30

Data from the National Soft Drink Association.

Caffeine Content of Some Chocolate Products

	MG Caffeine
Chocolate	
Baker's baking chocolate, unsweetened, 1 oz.	25
Baker's German sweet, 1 oz.	8
Baker's semi-sweet, 1 oz.	13
Baker's chocolate chips, 1/4 cup	13
Baker's German sweet chocolate chips, 1/4 cup	15
Cadbury chocolate bar, 1 oz.	15
Chocolate milk, 8 oz.	8
Desserts	
Jell-O Pudding Pops, chocolate	2
Jell-O Chocolate Mousse	6
Jell-O Chocolate Fudge Mousse	12
Beverages	
3 heaping teaspoons chocolate powder mix	8
2 tablespoons chocolate syrup	5
1 envelope hot cocoa mix	5

Data from Anne de Planter Bowes, *Bowes and Church's Food Values of Portions Commonly Used* (Philadelphia: Lippincott, 1989), pp. 261–2.

your metabolic rate and release stored fat to be burned as energy, although it is questionable as to whether it truly makes any difference during a diet. Diet aid manufacturers used to include caffeine and phenylpropanolamine (PPA) in diet pills to make a substitute amphetaminelike preparation. Even though the molecular structure of PPA is nearly identical to amphetamine, it is not nearly as potent. The FDA has not permitted the use of caffeine in diet pills for many years because manufacturers of the pills could not produce any evidence of its efficacy.

Caffeine does increase the level of fatty acids in the blood and has been shown to boost the oxidation of these fuels. For this reason, endurance athletes have used caffeine for years to promote the burning of fat and the sparing of muscle glycogen. But several recent caffeine studies don't support the long-held contention that caffeine spares glycogen stores to a significant extent—an effect that could help endurance athletes such as marathon runners to avoid running out of energy. But prerace caffeine can stave off feelings of fatigue and boost alertness.

The conversion of fat to energy is about 30 percent more efficient when caffeine is consumed prior to exercise. While the body burns fat, it reduces its reliance on glycogen, glucose, and amino acids, so blood sugar levels remain higher for longer. But even sedentary people can reap the mental benefits of caffeine. That is why coffee is popular among students, computer programmers, and think-tankers.

COFFEE'S CLEAN BILL OF HEALTH

Coffee has been given a clean bill of health by the following national health organizations:

- American Academy of Family Physicians
- American Cancer Society
- American Medical Association
- Association of Women's Health
- Framingham Heart Study
- International Food Information Council
- National Academy of Science
- National Research Council on Diet and Health
- Obstetric and Neonatal Nurses
- The Centers for Disease Control
- National Cancer Institute
- U.S. Food and Drug Administration
- U.S. Surgeon General

During the past two decades, coffee research has focused on the health aspects of caffeine consumption. The U.S. Food and Drug Administration (FDA) classified caffeine as Generally Recognized as Safe (GRAS) in 1958. Even sodas infused with caffeine got a passing grade when a recent scientific review found no evidence that the use of caffeine in carbonated beverages renders those products injurious to health.

The latest investigations of caffeine have concluded that moderate consumption poses no health risks to otherwise healthy adults. What is moderate consumption? Studies indicate that up to 300 milligrams of caffeine a day—equal to the caffeine in about three cups of regular brewed coffee—is safe. This depends, however, on one's tolerance to the compound and can vary depending on the day and whether caffeine is consumed in coffee or other beverages. People taking certain medications, those who are pregnant or breast-feeding, and those with caffeine sensitivity or health problems should consult with their physician before they consume caffeinated beverages.

GUARANÁ—THE AMAZON'S ALTERNATIVE TO COFFEE

Guaraná is an herb from the Amazon jungle whose unique properties were first introduced to the rest of the world by the tribe who gave the plant its name—the Guaranis. The active ingredient in guaraná is called guaranine, similar to caffeine, which is found in the seeds. Legend has it that the first guaraná plant sprouted from the buried eye of an infant god worshipped by the Guaranis. When you consider that the Guaranis require a great deal of stamina and endurance—to hunt for food and defend themselves from neighboring tribes—it's little wonder they invest spiritual significance in a plant providing that kind of staying power. Today, people the world over use guaraná powder and extract for much the same reason, to help them boost endurance and stay awake and alert.

In Europe, guaraná was first marketed as an alternative treatment for overall health, and the powder was and still is sold in health food shops. Although some retailers promote it as an aphrodisiac, there is not much evidence to support such a claim. More recently, guaraná has been used in "smart" drinks for people who want extra mental focus and cerebral energy. These drinks—most notably choline cocktails—provide a quick energy boost for those who need to use their brainpower for extended periods of time. Guaraná syrup is used for the manufacture of carbonated soft drinks, which are very popular in Brazil. Most energy drink manufacturers in the United States use guaraná that has been standardized for its caffeine content. This allows them to provide a measured dose of caffeine in their products— usually about the same as found in a cup of regular brewed coffee. Guaraná soda pop is ubiquitous in Brazil and is available in the United States at Latin American groceries.

CAFFEINE AND ATHLETIC PERFORMANCE

Professional athletes have consistently used caffeine to aid performance, especially during late afternoon workouts or as a means of getting "psyched up" for competition. At the cellular level, caffeine enhances neuromuscular transmission and improves skeletal muscle contractility. This is evident in tests that reveal reduced reaction times to a stimulus. Further research is needed before clear conclusions can be drawn regarding caffeine's effects on neuromuscular function and high-intensity exercise performance. Initially, researchers thought that caffeine improved endurance and performance by stimulating a greater use of fat for energy so that less of the stored energy (glycogen) in your muscles was burned.

Caffeine Can Tarnish Olympic Gold

The International Olympic Committee sets a limit on caffeine in urine tests corresponding to about four to five cups of coffee drunk in about thirty minutes. The IOC allows an upper limit of 12 mcg/ml of urine tested. Over a two- to three-hour period, a dose of 100 milligrams of caffeine results in a urine concentration of 1.5 mcg/ml. So, for example, if in a three-hour period you took 800 milligrams of caffeine (five to seven cups of strong coffee) you could exceed the legal dose. Depending on the individual, a range of 100 to 300 milligrams of caffeine has a stimulant effect. A dose of 2.3 mg/lb of body weight provides a stimulant effect yet is still legal according to the IOC rules. So the recommended legal dose for a 100-pound (45-kilogram) person would be 225 milligrams. This recommended legal dose, however, might not be enough to significantly improve performance by saving the energy in your muscles. To improve your endurance performance, you would have to take in so much caffeine that you would come close to exceeding the legal limit. This is risky business for athletes who want all the benefits of caffeine without the downside—being disqualified from competition and perhaps even losing an Olympic medal.

Caffeine is not for all athletes. For those who are extremely sensitive to its effects, it can cause headaches, nausea, and muscle tremors. Excessive caffeine intake can lead to dehydration, especially in hot weather. Not only do caffeine-sensitive athletes run the risk of negative reactions to the drug, they also risk losing the opportunity to compete. The current list of drugs banned by the International Olympic Committee (IOC) contains more than forty different stimulants, including caffeine. Because caffeine is a common ingredient in beverages, foods, and over-the-counter medications, its use is permitted by the IOC, but only in limited amounts. The IOC allows an upper limit of 12 micrograms (mcg) per milliliter (mL) of urine tested. Over a two-to-three-hour period, a dose of 100 milligrams (mg) of caffeine results in a urine concentration of 1.5 mcg/mL. A dose of 2.3 mg/lb of body weight provides a stimulant effect yet is still legal according to the IOC rules.

Many athletes can consume caffeine at levels equivalent to two to four cups of regular coffee without experiencing harsh side effects. Recent research suggests that the phytochemicals in coffee may exert a protective effect against colon cancer, so drinking coffee to boost endurance, alertness, and performance could have additional benefits.

DEBUNKING COFFEE MYTHS

An overwhelming body of research evidence has demonstrated that low-to-moderate caffeine intake does not increase the risk of or contribute to:

- Any type of human cancer
- Complications in pregnancy, adversity to fetus, infertility
- Breast disease
- Osteoporosis in adults (assuming adequate daily calcium intake)
- Cardiovascular diseases. Since caffeine increases athletic performance and endurance, caffeinated drinks may actually protect against heart disease.
- High blood pressure. Any caffeine-induced rise in blood pressure is short-lived, and generally is less than is experienced when climbing a stairway.
- Drug abuse. Caffeine use does not contribute to the destructive personal and criminal behavior seen with addictive drugs. In fact, coffee

has a beneficial effect on people's lives. A major study has found fewer suicides among coffee drinkers than those who abstained from the black brew.

Coffee even has one interesting side effect that may interest couples trying to conceive a child: There are studies that suggest drinking a cup of coffee prior to sexual intercourse can cause sperm to become more active in some men—and slow sperm is one of the leading causes of male infertility. Other studies contradict this finding. Before you stampede to the nearest Starbuck's, however, make sure you also ingest enough zinc—at least fifteen milligrams each day. Zinc (oysters are loaded with the mineral) plays an important role in testosterone synthesis and sperm production. Make mine an oyster latte, please.

CANCER

According to the American Cancer Society, "Available information does not suggest a recommendation against the moderate use of coffee. There is no indication that caffeine, a natural component of both coffee, tea, cocoa, and chocolate, is a risk factor in human cancer." A number of large international studies have found no relationship between coffee consumption and cancer risk. In fact, several recent studies have found that drinking coffee may lower the risk of developing colorectal cancer. Researchers at Boston's Harvard School of Public Health reviewed 17 studies on coffee drinking and health effects and discovered that study participants who drank four or more cups daily cut their risk of developing colorectal cancer by nearly 25 percent. They speculate that coffee contains compounds that accelerate peristalsis (smooth muscle contractions in the colon) and reduce the amount of time the interior intestine walls are exposed to carcinogens.

PREGNANCY

Researchers have long wondered if caffeine consumption could cause birth defects or reduce fertility rates. What is known is that caffeine does cause fetal malformations in rats, when ingested at rates equivalent to the amount contained in seventy cups of coffee a day. Human data is scant, as experimentation on humans is not feasible. In any case moderation in caffeine ingestion seems to be a prudent recommendation for pregnant women. The FDA has stated that caffeine does not adversely affect reproduction in humans, although the agency continues to preach moderation during pregnancy. However, three major studies involving more than 15,000 women found no birth defects associated with caffeine consumption even among the heaviest coffee drinkers. Similarly, other human studies continue to support the conclusion that moderate consumption of caffeine does not predispose expectant mothers to spontaneous abortion or preterm delivery, or the fetus to low birth weight. Research from the Centers for Disease Control and Prevention, Harvard Medical School, and the University of California at Berkeley show that moderate caffeine consumption does not reduce a woman's chance of becoming pregnant. A recent study found a weak link between sudden infant death syndrome (SIDS) and caffeine consumption by the mother, which reinforces the recommendation for moderation—and to be safe—abstinence.

OSTEOPOROSIS

Osteoporosis is a skeletal disease characterized by a decrease in bone density and the development of thin and brittle bones, prone to fracture. While it is not exclusively a women's disease, osteoporosis occurs most frequently in women. A 1984 National Institutes of Health (NIH) Consensus Report rejected caffeine as a risk factor for osteoporosis, emphasizing instead the importance of women building bone mass during their teenage years. A 1994 NIH consensus statement on optimum calcium intake does not mention caffeine among the factors that adversely affect calcium balance and induce loss of bone mass. Risk factors that contribute to osteoporosis include very low calcium and very high protein consumption, smoking, poor exercise habits, age, being Asian or Caucasian, low weight, and low estrogen levels. Several recent well-controlled studies have concluded that consuming moderate amounts of caffeine does not increase a woman's risk of osteoporosis. A Penn State Medical School study found that a lifetime consumption of caffeine, up to 800 mg/day (8+ cups of coffee), had no effect on bone density in 188 postmenopausal women. Health experts generally recommend that women who consume large amounts of caffeine—i.e., five cups or more a day—drink one glass of skim milk per day or take a calcium supplement to offset any possible caffeine-induced calcium losses. Most researchers agree that caffeine intake is not a significant risk factor for osteoporosis if—and that's the important word—people consume adequate calcium. If you follow the Ultimate Ratio plan and take a calcium/magnesium supplement each day, there is probably no need to worry about the caffeine-induced loss of calcium.

BREAST CANCER

A worldwide investigation of 100,000 deaths due to breast cancer found no relationship between caffeine intake and the development of this disease. Research has also shown that caffeine intake is not related to the development of fibrocystic breast disease (FBD), a condition of benign fibrous lumps in the breast, although there is some suggestion that caffeine may aggravate this condition. The American Medical Association's Council on Scientific Affairs and the National Cancer Institute have published reports stating there is no link between caffeine intake and the incidence of FBD. The American Cancer Society's *Guidelines on Diet, Nutrition and Cancer* states that caffeine is not a risk factor in human cancer. The National Academy of Sciences' National Research Council reports there is no persuasive evidence linking caffeine to any type of cancer.

CARDIOVASCULAR DISEASE

Evidence linking coffee consumption to the risk of coronary heart disease is weak and inconsistent. A 1989 report from the ongoing Framingham Heart Study examined all potential links between caffeine intake and cardiovascular disease, and found no harmful effects from drinking coffee. A recent Harvard University study confirmed this report, concluding that caffeine intake does not significantly raise the risk of coronary heart disease or stroke. Another Harvard study, which measured the coffee consumption of more than 85,000 female nurses for ten years, concluded that women who drink six or more cups of coffee a day may find themselves feeling a bit jumpy, but they are probably not increasing their risk for heart disease. After accounting for other heart disease risk factors, such as smoking, the researchers found no association between atherosclerosis and the consumption of either caffeinated or decaffeinated coffee or chocolate or colas. These findings contradict a number of earlier investigations that found a slight association between coffee and heart disease risk. Speculation about the possible link between heart disease and coffee drinking has focused on the brew's reputed ability to raise serum cholesterol levels. But the Harvard researchers say that this problem is seen mainly in people who drink large amounts of *unfiltered* coffee. Using paper filters appears to eliminate the chemicals suspected as being responsible for the cholesterol-raising effect.

HYPERTENSION

Consuming caffeine does not cause long-term hypertension or a persistent increase in blood pressure, except in a small subset of the elderly unaccustomed to caffeine. Some caffeine-sensitive people may experience a transient rise in blood pressure, usually not lasting more than a few hours. Studies show that a caffeine-induced rise in blood pressure is modest, usually less than that normally experienced when climbing stairs. Those with high blood pressure should consult their physician about caffeine intake.

Caffeine and Blood Pressure in Older Hypertensive Patients. Israeli researchers recently studied the effects of caffeine in young and old people. They found that caffeine can significantly increase blood pressure in a subset of older patients with hypertension, but not in younger hypertensives. Researchers monitored blood pressure changes in twenty-three adults with mild to moderate hypertension after the patients consumed 250 milligrams of caffeine powder dissolved in water. None of the adult participants were regular coffee drinkers, and all abstained from foods and products containing caffeine for two to three weeks before the study began. Thirteen of the subjects experienced a significant increase in blood pressure during the six hours following caffeine ingestion. People who responded adversely had a mean age of 58 years; those who had no pressure-raising effect from the caffeinated drink had a mean age of 44.5 years. Although studies of long-time caffeine intake indicate that people develop a tolerance to the blood pressure-raising effects of caffeine over time, short-term studies like this one indicate that the acute effects of caffeine, especially in elderly people, can be extremely significant.

CAFFEINE AND KIDS

Caffeine in small to moderate doses does not have any harmful affect on children's behavior, according to a recent analysis by researchers at the Universities of Chicago and Colorado. In fact, parents participating in a study of caffeine and theophylline (a compound commonly taken by children with asthma, and a close chemical cousin of caffeine), reported their kids behaved *better* after taking small doses of these compounds. Researchers at the NIH have concluded there is no difference in the way children and adults handle caffeine. These studies have shown that caffeine-containing foods and beverages do not have an effect on hyperactivity or the attention span of children. Parents should use common sense in deciding how much caffeine-containing foods or beverages they give their children, as with many foods. Consuming a caffeinated soft drink after a workout can deplete small amounts of minerals, including potassium and sodium. When it comes to calcium loss, the same cautions that apply to adults apply to children—perhaps even more so. Although most research concludes that caffeine consumption causes no significant loss of calcium in adults (provided they consume calcium-rich

U.S. Coffee Trivia

- On a typical day, approximately 49 percent of Americans drink coffee.
- On a per capita basis, men drink more coffee than women (1.7 cups per day vs. 1.5 cups).
- Coffee drinkers consume on average 3.3 cups of coffee per day.
- Thirty-seven percent of coffee drinkers drink their coffee black, while 63 percent add a sweetener and/or creaming agent.
- Regular coffee accounts for 87 percent of all coffee consumed; instant (soluble) coffee accounts for 13 percent.
- Fifty-seven percent of all coffee is consumed at breakfast; 34 percent between meals; and 13 percent at all other meals.
- Market research reveals that women are more excited than men about coffee varieties currently available and a higher proportion of women feel that drinking coffee is a good way to relax.
- Studies have shown that individuals who consume caffeine may increase their memory and improve reasoning powers; several tests indicated that they scored higher grades on motor skill tests, enhanced reaction times, and improved auditory and visual vigilance as opposed to noncaffeine consumers.
- When it comes to buying coffee for consumption at home, women are more price-conscious than men.

Coffee and Cholesterol—Should You Worry?

Much has been made in the press recently about coffee's ability to raise blood cholesterol levels. Men and women who drink filtered coffee exhibited no changes in blood cholesterol levels. Coffee filters effectively remove the diterpenes (cafestol and kahweol) in coffee—chemicals that raise cholesterol levels. People who drink coffee made by the French press method, however, display a host of unhealthy biochemical changes. For example, levels of one liver enzyme (alanine aminotransferase) can double in people who drink unfiltered coffee. This enzyme serves as a marker of potential liver damage. Fortunately, coffee drinkers experience enzyme elevations that are usually far less than in persons with liver disease. Moreover, the rise in liver enzymes is transient; most people adapt to such coffee intake after six months, the enzyme levels tending to normalize thereafter. Researchers have also observed a sharp, transitory rise in serum triglyceride levels among the men and women drinking French-pressed coffee. Like the liver-enzyme changes, however, the triglycerides fell as the study progressed. By the end of twenty-four weeks, their concentrations had already returned to levels recorded before the start of the study. Of far greater concern, however, are increases in levels of low-density-lipoprotein (LDL) cholesterol in volunteers drinking the pressed beverage. An increase in LDL cholesterol, a risk factor for heart disease, might over a lifetime elevate an individual's chance of developing coronary disease. Unfortunately, the elevation in LDL concentrations shows no sign of diminishing with time. Most espresso drinkers don't have to worry about large increases in LDL cholesterol levels owing to the small size of espresso cups. Instant coffee drinkers need not worry either, because all of the instant (regular and decaffeinated brands) tested thus far contain only trace quantities of the diterpenes in unfiltered coffee. The diterpenes that raise LDL are not found in other hot beverages such as tea and cocoa. Tea contains flavonoids, phytochemicals that help reduce the buildup of artery-clogging plaque.

foods), children must consume such calcium-rich foods as legumes, soy beverages, green leafy vegetables, and skim milk products or take calcium supplements to offset caffeine-induced losses of the mineral. In a recent study, researchers gave a group of 13- to 18-year-olds an unsweetened caffeinated drink. Their urinary calcium output increased by 25 percent (to 20 mg/hour for three hours). When they drank caffeine plus sugar, their calcium loss increased to 30 mg/hour. Consuming one cola soft drink may cost a child as much as 120 milligrams of calcium. If a child consumes caffeinated beverages, it is vital that this deficit be replaced by calcium in the diet.

HOT COCOA: MORE THAN JUST A FOOD?

Hot cocoa—a time-honored and delicious drink that warms the tummy and soothes the soul—has recently come under suspicion of harboring marijuanalike drugs hidden away in its complex food chemistry. Analyzing cocoa, researchers have discovered that it does contain substances mimicking marijuana's effects. But are there enough of these compounds to get us high?

In previous and widely publicized studies, scientists reported that cocoa contains anandamide, a pleasure-inducing compound produced in the brain, and two other substances that amplify anandamide's psychoactive effects.

After analyzing milk and cocoa separately, researchers in Naples, Italy, confirm that both contain anandamide and other compounds that produce a drug high. But neither milk nor cocoa appears to contain enough of these substances to produce marijuanalike effects, they believe. Stomach acid destroys most of the compounds before they can be absorbed into the bloodstream, according to the researchers.

Two other researchers at the University of California at Irvine, who previously reported finding marijuana-related substances in cocoa, argue that the Italian research team failed to test the concentrations of all the compounds found in cocoa. Ultimately, both groups of researchers leave open the possibility that chocolate may contain addictive compounds. Pass the Nestlé, please.

CAFFEINE "ADDICTION"

People use the word "addiction" loosely to indicate that they are hooked on chocolate, coffee, jogging, or work. There is no evidence whatsoever that caffeine cravings are even remotely comparable to those associated with serious drugs of abuse. The pharmacological effects of caffeine are transient, usually passing within a few hours. Caffeine does not accumulate in the body over the course of time and is normally excreted within several hours of consumption. The half-life of caffeine is the time it takes to eliminate one half of consumed caffeine from the body. This varies among individuals, and is about three to four hours in healthy adults. Smoking accelerates the metabolism of caffeine, generally reducing the half-life to less than three hours. People who regularly consume caffeine may drink several cups of coffee in a few hours and notice little effect, whereas a person who isn't a regular caffeine consumer may feel some stimulant effect after just one serving.

Caffeine-sensitive people who feel any unpleasant side effects tend to limit their caffeine consumption. When regular caffeine consumption is abruptly discontinued, some people may experience withdrawal symptoms, such as headaches, fatigue, or drowsiness. These effects usually are temporary, lasting up to a day or so, and often can be avoided if caffeine cessation is gradual. Nearly all health experts agree that any discomfort caused by abruptly ceasing caffeine consumption can be avoided by progressively decreasing intake over a few days.

GREEN TEA

Green tea contains phytonutrients known as polyphenols, which act as powerful antioxidants. One cup of green tea usually contains about 300 to 400 milligrams of polyphenols, which provide powerful disease-fighting properties. In addition to exerting antioxidant activity on its own, green tea may expand the activity of antioxidant enzymes glutathione reductase, glutathione peroxidase, glutathione S-transferase, catalase, and quinone reductase in the small intestine, lungs, and liver. In animal studies, green tea extracts protected against UV-induced skin cancers, reducing cancer occurrence by up to 62 percent. Interestingly, the induction of skin tumors by UV radiation was significantly reduced by topical, but not oral, administration of purified green tea extracts.

A number of cancer studies have shown that green tea polyphenols inhibit cancer by blocking the formation of nitrosamines (carcinogenic amino acid-like compounds that form in the stomach) and by suppressing the activation of carcinogens in lung, breast, colon, and melanoma cancers. Green tea extracts have been shown to have inhibitory effects on the growth of mammary cancer cells by inhibiting the interaction of estrogen with its receptors in a manner similar to that of soy isoflavones.

Be careful not to drink your green tea too hot. Researchers have examined the effects of drinking very hot tea and have found that high temperatures were associated with increased stomach cancer risk. Drinking near-boiling hot tea increased the risk of cancer, supporting two earlier studies in which it was noted that very hot foods increased stomach and upper gastrointestinal tract cancers.

Dietary surveys in Japan reveal that people who consume three to six cups of green tea each day enjoy low rates of breast, colon, pancreatic, stomach, liver, lung, esophageal, and skin cancers. Green tea may prevent cancer by:

- Neutralizing cancer-causing agents;
- Protecting cells against mutations from carcinogens;
- Protecting cells against free radical damage;
- Protecting cells against radiation damage.

Studies have shown that green tea consumption also protects against cardiovascular disease in four ways, by:

- Reducing total cholesterol and elevating HDL cholesterol;
- Inhibiting abnormal clotting in blood vessels;
- Reducing high blood pressure;
- Inhibiting the oxidation of LDL cholesterol.

Green tea has also demonstrated an ability to reduce blood glucose levels, inhibit the growth of bacteria and viruses, boost fat burning, and act as a general antioxidant.

LAST BUT NOT LEAST—WATER

After oxygen, water is the most important "nutrient" in the body. Water comprises more than 70 percent of the body's tissues and functions as coolant, transport agent, solvent, and lubricant. Water is as vital to survival as it is essential to peak physical performance. Is it any wonder that I call it the drink of champions?

Ironically, the people who need to consume the most water—professional athletes—don't drink enough of it, while inactive designer water–lovers tend to drink more than they need. This observation has always amazed me. In my work with world-champion athletes in almost every major sport, invariably none of them consumed enough water until I began consulting with them.

In the ordinary American diet, most adults consume about two quarts of water a day, with two thirds coming from water and other beverages and the remainder coming from food. When you eat according to the Ultimate Ratio you will have no need to count the number of glasses of water you drink each day. A simple way to monitor the adequacy of your fluid intake is to monitor the color of your urine: Pale-yellow to clear urine throughout the day indicates that you are consuming enough water to satisfy your body's need for fluid.

There are people with such medical conditions as urinary tract infections and kidney stones who could benefit from consciously increasing their fluid intake beyond the recommended six to eight ounces of fluid a day. Other medical conditions, such as low blood levels of potassium, require that people restrict their water consumption. *Check with a physician to determine if there is any reason why you should increase or decrease your fluid consumption.* You've already learned that a high-protein diet can dehydrate your body by overloading it with ammonia and other nitrogen-related compounds. But many Americans may be literally drinking themselves to dehydration simply by drinking too many alcoholic drinks. Alcohol acts as a diuretic, causing the body to lose water through increased urination. According to published surveys, many people are aware that most health experts recommend drinking six to eight ounces of fluid each day, but nearly 50 percent admitted to not drinking that amount.

Several studies report that consumption of caffeinated beverages can lead to water loss because the drug acts as a diuretic. While it is true that caffeine drinks can cause small losses of water and minerals, you can easily compensate for such losses by consuming a little extra water and using a multivitamin-mineral supplement.

Caffeinated beverages can improve sports performance and endurance and should not be avoided solely because of a mild diuretic effect. Athletes engaged in endurance events and those involved in sports that depend on quick reflexes and hand-eye coordination can benefit from using caffeinated drinks before competition. Simply drink an additional glass of water or sports drink just before or during physical activity and caffeine will pose no threat to your hydration status.

Each quart of sweat that you lose contains approximately 500–1,000 milligrams of sodium, 150–250 milligrams of potassium and about 500 milligrams of chloride. Since the Ultimate Ratio contains plenty of water-rich and mineral-dense foods, including fruits and vegetables, you will have an added measure of security that can help prevent dehydration due to alcohol and caffeine consumption.

Here's a simple rule of thumb: An active person who burns 2,000 calories per day will need 2,000 milliliters (about 2 quarts) of water or fluid every day; a couch potato who burns 1,500 calories requires about 1.5 quarts (6 cups) of water. Add one additional cup of water to that amount if you drink one or two cups of coffee or enjoy a glass of wine each evening. Add two cups if you drink between two to four cups of coffee or two or more alcoholic beverages.

An athlete who weighs 160 pounds and loses just 3.2 pounds during exercise will experience a reduced performance capability. Athletes who run at a six-minute-mile pace in hot, humid environments can expect to lose fluid at a rate of approximately 2.0–2.5 liters per hour. I recommend measuring your body weight before and after each training session to get an idea of how much fluid you can expect to lose during a particular training session.

8

REVENGE OF THE NERDS

USING NOOTROPICS TO MAKE A MIND-BODY CONNECTION

N erds got the jump on professional athletes by discovering how to use the power of nootropics to boost psychic energy, mental focus, and concentration.

Nootropics?

Yes, nootropics (pronounced nū-tropé-icks). In the late 1980s, computer programmers and hackers beat athletes to the punch—in this case, the punch was a "choline cocktail"—by learning how to use "smart drinks," the street name for nootropic beverages. Recently, Wall Street traders and commodities brokers learned about the mind-boosting effects of these beverages and began using them in their fast-paced jobs. And now you can learn how to use them—on the field, at the office, or in the classroom.

SMART NUTRIENTS FOR PEAK PERFORMANCE

What are nootropics? Think of them as nutrients found in specific foods, dietary supplements, and commercial smart drinks that boost mental focus, memory, thinking, learning, alertness, and reaction time to a stimulus.

Smart nutrients occur naturally in ordinary foods. For example, fish has long been referred to as brain food—for good reason. Besides the fact that they travel in schools, fish contain a compound called DMAE—

dimethylaminoethanol—a smart nutrient that enhances mental activity. DMAE helps the brain synthesize acetylcholine, involved in boosting concentration, enhancing memory, and controlling muscular movement. DMAE is also available as a nutritional supplement.

Some smart nutrients protect brain cells from oxidation and premature aging. Still others can slow down the progression of such conditions as Alzheimer's and senility or even improve cognition in people who already have them. Athletes are interested in using smart drinks to connect the brain to brawn. That's because these drinks help supercharge the mind-body connection, which can put an athlete in the zone of peak performance. Martina Navratilova, Ivan Lendl, and many other world champions have used my smart drinks to outsmart formidable foes. Now you can use them to do the same.

How do smart nutrients work their mind-body magic?

Your brain cells speak to one another and to the rest of the body by releasing communicative chemicals called neurotransmitters. Neurotransmitters control a variety of the body's functions, including memory, mental energy, intelligence, sex drive, sleep, appetite, mood, and physical performance.

The body makes four important neurotransmitters from the amino acids found in the Ultimate Ratio food groups.

As your body digests whole protein from Ultimate Ratio foods, making amino acids, the blood shuttles these amino acids to organs and tissues, including muscles (for growth, maintenance, and energy) and the nerves and brain (for neurotransmitter synthesis). Four key neurotransmitters control intelligence, movement, memory, alertness, weight loss, sexuality, sleep, and mood. Your level of physical and mental performance depends on the levels of neurotransmitters your body makes each day.

Smart Nutrient (Food Source)	Neurotransmitter
Choline, DMAE, betaine (Fish, legumes, soy foods, beets)	Acetylcholine
L-phenylalanine, L-tyrosine (Soy foods, seafood, legumes, meats)	Dopamine and norepinephrine
L-tryptophan (Soy foods, bananas, milk, potato, pumpkin)	Serotonin

The Ultimate Ratio contains the ideal foods to help the body make the four vital neurotransmitters that supercharge the maximum mind-body connection.

A number of vitamins and minerals are also required for promoting the synthesis of brain neurotransmitters. Unlike amino acids, these nutrients do not compete with each other for entry into the brain. Vitamin C, for example, has its own special "pump" in the brain to regulate the entry of this important smart nutrient. Other vitamins are transported to the brain by special carrier molecules. To make the mood- and sleep-regulating neurotransmitter serotonin from the amino acid L-tryptophan, the brain uses vitamin B_3 and vitamin B_6. The brain requires vitamins B_3, B_6, and C, folic acid, and the minerals copper, iron, and zinc to transform the amino acids L-phenylalanine and L-tyrosine into dopamine and norepinephrine. Vitamins B_1, B_5, B_6, and C, and the minerals zinc and calcium are required for acetylcholine production.

THE SUPER CHOLINE COCKTAIL

What do Wall Street traders, commodity brokers, world-champion athletes, computer programmers, and entertainers have in common? They are the people most familiar with my Super Choline Cocktail. But even though tennis professionals have used it to win world championships, and entertainers use it to boost mental energy, focus, and creativity, most people outside of these professions have not yet heard about this powerful mind-body beverage. Whether you spearhead a hostile takeover of a corporation, face a fierce opponent on center court, perform in front of millions of TV viewers, write computer code for Microsoft Corporation, cram for an MIT mid-term, or simply dance the night away at a local club, a choline cocktail may be just what the doctor ordered.

The Ultimate Ratio choline cocktail contains such mind-body nutrients as choline, DMAE, and guaraná to help achieve mental focus and think faster and more accurately. You don't have to be an elite athlete to reap the rewards of these mind-body nutrients. Anyone who needs extended mental and physical energy can benefit from using a choline cocktail. Many people use it in place of their morning coffee and before a mentally or physically demanding event.

You can make the choline cocktail in your own kitchen—all you need is

Super Choline Cocktail

1,500 mg choline	1,000 mcg cobalamin (vitamin B_{12})
100 mg DMAE	300 mcg biotin
100 mcg chromium picolinate	400 mcg folic acid
60 mg ginkgo biloba	1,000 mg vitamin C
1.5 mg thiamin (vitamin B_1)	15 mg coenzyme Q_{10}
1.9 mg riboflavin (vitamin B_2)	100 mg caffeine (from guaraná)
20 mg niacinamide (vitamin B_3)	400 IU vitamin E
100 mg pantothenic acid (vitamin B_5)	8 ounces cold fruit juice (any kind)
2 mg pyridoxine (vitamin B_6)	

If supplements are in tablet form, crush them until they are the consistency of fine powder, using a food processor or a mortar and pestle. If supplements are in capsule form, open capsule and empty contents into a container to which crushed tablets have been added.

Put the powder in a blender with 2 to 4 ice cubes and pour in the cold juice.

Blend until smooth in a blender or food processor and serve immediately.

NOTE: This drink should not be used by young children or pregnant or breast-feeding women, people with any health condition or disease, including high blood pressure or heart disease, or those wishing to eliminate caffeine from their diet.

a blender. If you don't have the time or inclination to make your own, you can purchase a premixed choline cocktail from vitamin shops and natural food stores.

For convenience, I recommend the Twin Laboratories *Choline Cocktail,* which is cheaper than making the drink from individual ingredients and also tastes much better because the choline, which has a bitter and often fishy flavor, has been microencapsulated to render it tasteless.

If you don't want to use a choline cocktail, you may want to focus on eating choline-rich foods. The ordinary American diet contains between 500 and 1,000 milligrams of choline. A list of the best sources of this mind-muscle nutrient is given in the table on page 126.

Choline and DMAE are smart nutrients that help boost the brain's supply of acetylcholine, a neurotransmitter that regulates bodily movements. In addition to these two nutrients, acetylcholine synthesis also requires vitamin B_5 (pantothenic acid), vitamin B_6 (pyridoxine) and vitamin C (ascorbic acid). Vitamin B_5 can be found in brewer's yeast, corn, lentils, lobster, meats, peas, soybeans, sunflower seeds, wheat germ, and whole grains. Vitamin B_6 is found in avocados, bananas, carrots, lentils, salmon, shrimp, soy foods, and

Choline-Rich Foods	(MG)
Wheat germ (½ cup)	2,829
Peanuts (½ cup)	1,113
Peanut butter (½ cup)	966
Calf's liver (3.5 ounces)	850
Ham (3.5 ounces)	800
Lamb chops (3.5 ounces)	753
Whole-wheat flour (½ cup)	613
White rice (1.2 cup)	586
Trout (3.5 ounces)	580
Beef (eye round; 3.5 ounces)	453
Whole egg (1 large)	394
White flour (½ cup)	346
Pecans (½ cup)	333

NOTE: Other choline-rich foods include soy foods, cabbage, cauliflower, caviar, egg yolks, garbanzo beans, lentils, and split peas.

white albacore tuna. Vitamin C-rich foods include broccoli, Brussels sprouts, cabbage, citrus fruits, peppers, and tomatoes.

Crossing the Blood-Brain Barrier

Mother Nature designed the blood-brain barrier (BBB) to protect the brain against the onslaught of potentially harmful chemicals we eat, drink, and breathe each day. The BBB (actually a series of small blood vessels and special cells that support and nourish brain neurons, called glial cells) regulates the entry of smart nutrients and drugs into your brain.

Getting specific amino acids to cross the BBB in sufficient quantities to boost mental performance presents a problem simply because the BBB is so selective. So how can an athlete who wants to make a mind-body connection make sure that enough of a particular amino acid crosses the BBB to stimulate the synthesis of its corresponding neurotransmitter? The answer involves learning just a few biochemical tricks:

• **Brute force:** Whenever you significantly increase the ratio of one amino acid over the others, you saturate the BBB's transport mechanisms that lock on to that specific nutrient and carry it into the brain. The result is that you will get more of one smart nutrient into the brain simply by over-

Smart Drugs in the Brain

Here are the four vital neurotransmitters—your brain's own smart drugs—that help determine your level of mental and physical performance. The Ultimate Ratio plan provides the smart nutrients your body needs to synthesize optimal levels of these neurotransmitters:

Acetylcholine

Acetylcholine is the most abundant neurotransmitter in the body. It is responsible for helping nerves talk to muscles. It helps the body perform a variety of "housekeeping" functions, such as blood flow, heartbeat, and sweating. Acetylcholine also helps control muscle tone, learning, and primitive drives and emotions. Low acetylcholine levels can contribute to forgetfulness and lack of concentration and may cause you to be a light sleeper. The body synthesizes acetylcholine from the smart nutrients choline, lecithin, DMAE, and betaine, with the help of vitamins C, B_5, and B_6, along with the minerals zinc and calcium.

Norepinephrine

Norepinephrine stimulates the release of stored body fat and helps control the release of endocrine hormones (e.g., those concerned with appetite, fertility, sex drive, and metabolism). It also helps regulate learning and memory. Norepinephrine is synthesized from two amino acids (L-phenylalanine and L-tyrosine, found in such high-protein foods as soy, turkey, seafood, and beef). The body uses vitamins C, B_3, and B_6, along with zinc and copper to make this neurotransmitter.

Dopamine

Dopamine helps regulate muscular movement, sex drive, tissue growth and repair, and immune system function. It also stimulates the pituitary gland to secrete growth hormone, which builds muscle and burns fat. Dopamine is chemically related to norepinephrine and L-dopa (a prescription drug used to treat Parkinson's disease), and, like norepinephrine, is synthesized from the amino acids L-phenylalanine and L-tyrosine.

Serotonin

Serotonin plays an important role in blood clotting, stimulating a strong heartbeat, initiating sleep, fighting depression (prescription drugs that treat depression raise the brain's levels of serotonin) and in causing migraine headaches in susceptible individuals (due to its ability to constrict blood vessels and/or cause them to spasm). Serotonin is synthesized from the amino acid L-tryptophan. Serotonin serves as a precursor for the pineal hormone melatonin, which helps regulate the body's sleep-wake cycles and immune system. Rich sources of L-tryptophan include bananas, milk, turkey, soy foods, pumpkin, and sunflower seeds.

Selected Sources of L-tryptophan

Food	Amount	MG
Spirulina (nutritional supplement)	3.5 oz	929
Pumpkin (roasted)	1 oz	164
Milk (whole, low-fat, or skim))	1 cup	115
Sunflower seeds (dried)	1 oz	99
Potato, baked with skin	1 medium	77
Tomato soup made with skim milk	1 cup	77
Shredded wheat	1 oz	49
Seaweed, kelp (kombu, tangle)	3.5 oz	48
Turnip greens (boiled)	½ cup	48
Collard greens (boiled)	1 cup	27

feeding it relative to all others. Taking individual supplementary amino acids several hours distant from meals will help them cross the BBB.

• **Eat foods rich in phenylalanine and tyrosine:** If you want to increase the amount of neurotransmitters norepinephrine and dopamine in the brain, consume seafood that is rich in L-phenylalanine and L-tyrosine (these amino acids serve as building blocks for the synthesis of norepinephrine, which will wake up your brain). White albacore tuna fish packed in water makes, a healthy choice for accomplishing this feat (see Power-Packed Tuna Salad, page 185).

• **Tryptophan-loading:** Using this clever trick, you can get L-tryptophan into your brain to help get a good night's sleep before an important match. Here's how it works: The BBB tightly regulates L-tryptophan's entry into the brain. But if you consume a carbohydrate-rich snack that contains soy or skim milk and bananas (all rich in L-tryptophan) and honey (for carbohydrate), you can trick the brain into welcoming L-tryptophan with open arms. That's because insulin, the hormone secreted by the pancreas in response to protein and carbohydrate consumption, clears a path for L-tryptophan's entry across the BBB.

THE ULTIMATE RATIO SMART NUTRIENT LIST

Below is a selection of smart nutrients and compounds most often found in dietary supplement formulas designed to make a mind-body connection, boost mental performance, and slow down mental deterioration due to drug use, environmental pollution, and ordinary aging.

When it comes to the gray matter of the brain, nothing is black and white. Smart nutrients, like drugs, have a wide variety of primary (intended) and secondary (undesirable) effects. *Always check with a physician before taking these or any other supplements.*

GINKGO BILOBA

Ginkgo biloba is a smart nutrient found in the leaves of the oldest surviving species of tree known. Leaf extracts from the ginkgo biloba tree have been used by Chinese medicine for thousands of years, mainly as a tonic to improve blood flow to the brain and enhance mental alertness. Human studies have revealed that gingko increases brain metabolism by promoting the synthesis of adenosine triphosphate, or ATP (the most important energy-producing compound in the body); it improves the brain's ability to metabolize glucose, thereby increasing the production of ATP and reducing blood-clotting time in the brain. Gingko also acts as an antioxidant, and several studies have shown it to improve short-term memory loss in the elderly. Asian physicians have prescribed gingko for people with symptoms of reduced blood flow to the brain and extremities.

Dosage commonly used: Most ginkgo biloba supplements contain an extract standardized to a 24 percent concentration (look for this number on the package label). At this strength, the typical dosage is between 120 and 150 milligrams per day divided over three equal doses.

PHYTOESTROGENS

These are hormonelike plant and fruit extracts that play a key role in maximum mental performance. Phytoestrogens derived from soy foods, whole grains, and legumes may have a beneficial effect on memory because some can mimic the memory-enhancing effects of the body's own natural hormone, estrogen. Estrogen supports healthy brain function and memory (both men and women make estrogen from ordinary cholesterol). Researchers at the McGill University Menopause Clinic uncovered estrogen's importance in maintaining memory by testing verbal memory in young women before and after they were treated for uterine tumors. The women's estrogen levels plummeted after twelve weeks of chemotherapy, as did their scores on reading retention tests. But when researchers supplemented half of the group's regular therapy with estrogen, their performance promptly rebounded. Results of other studies suggest that women who take estrogen may lower their risk of Alzheimer's disease. The reasons are still unclear, but the hormone appears to support the development of certain brain neurons and boost the production of the neurotransmitter acetylcholine, which is involved in memory.

Dosage commonly used: Since taking estrogen may increase the risk of certain cancers, especially in women predisposed to breast cancer, drinking a phytoestrogen-rich soy cocktail daily, such as the Super Strawberry Shake (page 176), may provide all of the memory- and brain-boosting effects of estrogen without the dangerous side effects.

Phytoestrogen-Rich Foods

Soy foods	Lentils
Soy milk	Whole grains
Beans	Brown rice
Peas	

CAFFEINE

Caffeine (and related methylxanthine compounds found in tea, cocoa, and chocolate) is probably the best-known mind fitness nutrient in the world. Ironically, millions of coffee and tea lovers may be addicted more to the calming effects of caffeine rather than to its stimulant properties. Coffee actually contains a number of opiate-related compounds that exert a mild heroinlike effect on the brain (decaf lovers obtain the same dose of these compounds, since they remain after decaffeination). Caffeine helps reduce typing errors, boosts mental alertness, energy, and the ability to do work even when fatigued. Caffeine blocks the effect of a brain-calming chemical, adenosine, and stimulates the release of norepinephrine, a neurotransmitter that stimulates mental function.

Dosage commonly used: Most healthy people can consume up to 300 milligrams per day (the approximate amount in three cups of brewed coffee) without any adverse health effects. Green tea, generally sold in health food stores, contains about half the caffeine of coffee per serving and also contains potent antioxidant smart nutrients called polyphenols, which protect against heart disease, stroke, and cancer.

Caffeine-Containing Foods

Coffee	Cocoa
Tea	Chocolate

VITAMIN B₁ (THIAMIN) AND B₂ (RIBOFLAVIN)

VITAMIN B_1 (THIAMIN) AND B_2 (RIBOFLAVIN)

These vitamins help control energy production from glucose in the brain and nervous system. They assist in the formation of the fatty acids that lend structural integrity to membranes of nerve cells (neurons) and participate in the synthesis of one memory-related brain neurotransmitter, acetylcholine. Avoid consuming raw fish, raw eggs, and large amounts of alcohol, since these foods destroy vitamin B_1; vitamin B_2 is destroyed by light and cooking.

Dosage commonly used: Most high-potency vitamin formulas on the market contain a daily dosage of between 10 and 50 milligrams each of thiamin and riboflavin.

Thiamin-Rich Foods

Brewer's yeast	Rice bran
Garbanzo beans	Rice, brown
Kidney (beef)	Salmon
Kidney beans	Soybeans
Liver (beef)	Sunflower seeds
Navy beans	Wheat germ
Pork	Whole-grain flour

Riboflavin-Rich Foods

Almonds	Chicken
Brewer's yeast	Kidney (beef)
Dairy products (cheese, milk, yogurt)	Wheat germ

VITAMIN B₃ (NIACINAMIDE)

Your brain and nervous system require optimal amounts of niacinamide to perform at maximum levels (the body can also convert the amino acid L-tryptophan into niacin; some authorities believe that up to two thirds of the body's daily requirement for the vitamin can be satisfied by L-tryptophan).

Dosage commonly used: Most high-potency vitamin formulas contain between 25 and 125 milligrams of niacinamide, the amount to be taken daily.

Niacinamide-Rich Foods

Beets	Salmon
Brewer's yeast	Sunflower seeds
Chicken	Swordfish
Fish (especially halibut)	Tuna (white albacore)
Peanuts	Turkey
Pork	Veal

VITAMIN B₅

This vitamin, pantothenic acid, participates in the synthesis of the brain neurotransmitter acetylcholine. It is particularly abundant in meat, fish, and legumes.

Dosage commonly used: Most high-potency vitamin formulas contain 100 to 500 milligrams of pantothenic acid, the recommended daily dosage.

Pantothenic Acid–Rich Foods

Brewer's yeast	Meats, all kinds
Cheese (blue)	Peanuts
Corn	Peas
Eggs	Soybeans
Lentils	Sunflower seeds
Liver (beef)	Wheat germ
Lobster	Whole-grain (wheat) flour

VITAMIN B$_6$

This vitamin, also called pyridoxine, assists in the transport and metabolism of the amino acids used by the brain to manufacture neurotransmitters involved in mental energy and memory. Chronic megadoses of this vitamin (1 to 6 grams per day) used to treat carpal tunnel syndrome have led, in a few cases, to vitamin toxicity (peripheral neuropathy), which disappeared once the dosage of B$_6$ was reduced.

Dosage commonly used: Most high-potency multi-vitamin formulas supply between 10 and 75 milligrams of vitamin B$_6$ per day. Certain conditions, such as pregnancy, oral contraceptive use, and increased protein intake, can increase your need for Vitamin B$_6$. Check with a physician before you take vitamin B$_6$ supplements.

Pyridoxine-Rich Foods

Avocados	Lentils
Bananas	Rice (brown)
Bran (wheat and rice)	Salmon
Brewer's yeast	Shrimp
Carrots	Soybeans
Filbert nuts	Sunflower seeds

CHOLINE AND LECITHIN

Choline and phosphatidyl choline (popularly known as lecithin) increase the brain's synthesis of acetylcholine, a neurotransmitter involved in memory, learning, and mental alertness. Peanuts, wheat germ, ham, trout, and calf's liver are rich sources of phosphatidyl choline; Brussels sprouts, oatmeal, soybeans, cabbage, cauliflower, kale, spinach, carrots, lettuce, and potatoes also contain appreciable amounts of choline chloride.

Dosage commonly used: Most memory-boosting supplement formulas on the market contain 1 to 1.5 grams of choline chloride or choline bitartrate. Choline, unlike amino acids, does not have to be taken on an empty stomach because no known nutrient competes with choline for absorption. See page 126 for a list of choline-rich foods.

DMAE (DIMETHYLAMINOETHANOL)

DMAE can increase the brain's production of acetylcholine. Recent studies have shown that DMAE can elevate mood, improve memory and learning, and even extend the life span of laboratory animals. Although DMAE is a nutrient found in small amounts in such seafood as sardines and anchovies, most smart nutrient formulas call for 50 to 100 milligrams, which requires the use of a DMAE supplement (DMAE is usually a component of most commercially prepared choline cocktails). DMAE has been used to treat learning disorders in children, especially in children with shortened attention spans and hyperactivity. The brain stimulant effect of DMAE develops slowly over a period of weeks, with no druglike letdown when discontinued.

Dosage commonly used: Smart nutrient users generally start with low doses of DMAE (100 per day), with a gradual buildup to 500+ mg per day. Overdosage can cause insomnia, headaches, and muscle tension. A physician should monitor people with epilepsy if they use DMAE. Those people who suffer from manic depression should avoid taking DMAE because it can intensify the depressive phase of this disease. DMAE is a volatile compound that should be stored in a cool, dark place. It is available in bulk powder form, liquid, and capsules.

DMAE-Rich Foods

Sardines   Anchovies

VITAMIN C

This vitamin is so important to maintaining brain health that the brain and central nervous system contain vitamin C "pumps" to maintain a high concentration of the vitamin. Brain cells have a high unsaturated fat content, which makes them susceptible to oxidation and damage from toxic atoms or molecules called free radicals. The brain requires high levels of vitamin C to prevent brain damage and premature aging. Studies have shown that students with higher vitamin C levels in their blood scored better on IQ tests than those with lower vitamin C blood levels. Vitamin C is required for the synthesis of acetylcholine and norepinephrine, two brain neurotransmitters involved in memory and learning.

Dosage commonly used: Many health professionals recommend between 250 and 1,000 milligrams of vitamin C daily (the less acidic form of vitamin C, calcium ascorbate, is widely available for those people with sensitive stomachs).

Vitamin C-Rich Foods

Black currants	Oranges
Broccoli	Papayas
Brussels sprouts	Peppers (green, sweet red, chili peppers)
Cabbage	Potatoes
Collard greens	Spinach
Grapefruit	Strawberries
Kalet	Tomatoes
Kiwi frui	Watercress
Lemons	

COENZYME Q_{10}

CoQ_{10} helps supply brain neurons with energy in the form of ATP, and its antioxidant properties help protect the brain's cell membranes. Tissue concentrations of CoQ_{10} are depleted under a variety of conditions, including stress, various kinds of illness, exposure to cold, drugs, and physical activity. You can find a small dose of this valuable nonvitamin nutrient in white albacore tuna (with spring water).

Dosage commonly used: No one has yet determined the amount of CoQ_{10} needed for optimal health (this amount will vary according to the individual), but published research reveals that daily dosages in the range of 10 to 120 milligrams are safe and effective.

Coenzyme Q_{10}-Rich Foods

Beef	Spinach
Peanuts	Tuna (white albacore)
Sardines	

VITAMIN B_{12} AND FOLIC ACID (OR FOLATE)

I've lumped these two vitamins together because of their similar functions. Vitamin B_{12} is unusual in that its only source in nature is synthesis by microorganisms. The vitamin is not found in plants except when contaminated by microbes. Vitamin B_{12} is found in meat, seafood (fish, clams, oysters, crabs), poultry, and, to a lesser extent, milk and dairy products. Vitamin B_{12} helps regulate carbohydrate and protein metabolism in the brain, promotes myelin synthesis in nerves (myelin is the protective fatty sheath surrounding nerve branches), and is indirectly involved in making choline available for neurotransmitter synthesis. Folic acid is required for the synthesis of memory molecules (such as ribonucleic acid, or RNA) in the brain. It also helps control protein metabolism in the brain and plays an essential role in the development of the nervous system in the fetus. Common food sources of folic acid include such leafy green vegetables as lettuce, spinach, kale, and collard greens, and fresh fruits. Vitamin B_6, another mind fitness nutrient discussed previously, is intimately involved in the metabolic roles played by vitamin B_{12} and folic acid.

Dosage commonly used: High-potency vitamin formulas generally contain between 500 and 1,000 micrograms of vitamin B_{12} and 100 to 800 mcg of folic acid. Recent research has shown that 400 to 800 milligrams of folic acid daily can prevent certain birth defects related to the central nervous system. Oral Vitamin B_{12} supplements are absorbed well even in the elderly, who may have an impaired ability to absorb this vitamin.

Folate-Rich Foods

Barley	Liver (calf's)
Beans (most types)	Oranges
Brewer's yeast	Peas
Endive	Rice (brown)
Fruits (almost all)	Soybeans
Garbanzo beans	Sprouts (alfalfa)
Leafy green vegetables (almost all)	Wheat germ
Lentils	

CHROMIUM PICOLINATE

This special form of the mineral chromium was developed and patented by scientists at the U.S. Department of Agriculture. Chromium helps the hormone insulin remove carbohydrate from the blood and get it into brain cells, where it can be metabolized for energy. The body may absorb chromium picolinate more efficiently than it does ordinary chromium.

Dosage commonly used: Recently published chromium picolinate studies have used 200 mcg per day in women. Some experts believe that weight lifters and other athletes of both sexes may need up to 400 mcg per day. Chromium picolinate is available in smart drinks, high-potency multivitamin–mineral formulas, and capsules that supply 200 mcg in each.

L-CARNITINE

Without this smart nutrient, your body can't burn fat. L-carnitine actually transports fat to the fat-burning furnace in each cell, the mitochondrion. While your body can manufacture a certain amount of L-carnitine each day, research has shown that certain conditions may deplete your body's supply of L-carnitine, such as aging, high fat consumption, exercise, stress, steroid use, illness, alcohol ingestion, high protein consumption, and glycogen (the storage form of carbohydrate) synthesis. A recently published research study also demonstrated that L-carnitine may act as an ergogenic (energy-giving) substance, improving endurance in trained athletes, most likely by stimulating the synthesis of the energy molecule, ATP.

Dosage commonly used: 250 to 1,000 milligrams per day.

9

THE ULTIMATE RATIO

QUESTIONS & ANSWERS

The world has no shortage of diet experts who are eager to tell you the healthiest way to eat for fitness, longevity, and permanent weight loss. Many of these so-called experts want you to eat according to your blood type, body type, or personality type. Others want you to shun carbohydrates or avoid eating foods that contain protein and carbohydrates in the same meal. All of these schemes lack the same important element: *scientific merit.* What they don't lack is a large audience, willing to blindly embrace them and even defend them. In the end, most fail miserably to deliver their promise of helping you achieve permanent fat loss, optimal health, and peak mental and physical performance. My readers and clients have always stayed far ahead of the rest of the world, nutritionally speaking, because my research has always been ahead of its time. If you aspire to win an Olympic Gold medal or win the finals at Wimbledon, or you have just been handed a diagnosis of cancer, heart disease, diabetes, or osteoporosis by your doctor, I am one person with whom you or your physician should consult. But since I am only one person, I cannot personally advise everyone who seeks my counsel. That's why I write diet, health, and fitness books. It allows me to "clone" myself to a certain degree and give my readers the benefit of my nutritional counsel. Of course, professional athletes need far more detail than I can possibly put in a book, but recreational and serious amateur athletes or kids and teens who aspire to become professional athletes can use my books to help them take a giant step toward achieving their goals.

I have received hundreds of questions about foods, fitness, fat loss, vitamins, minerals, cholesterol, and phytonutrients over the years. Here are my answers to the questions most frequently asked by my clients and readers.

What distinguishes the Ultimate Ratio plan from all other fat-loss plans?

The Ultimate Ratio plan is based on the most up-to-date scientific knowledge in food science and nutrition. It combines delicious and nutritious foods from the two healthiest diets in the world, the Mediterranean and Asian diets, and includes some very healthy foods and beverages such as chocolate, coffee, cocoa, wine, and beer that are often prohibited on diet plans. It helps control the body's glycogen levels, in a measured and scientific way, to help dieters achieve their fat-loss goals. It also emphasizes a new generation of scientifically formulated functional foods and drinks, based on soy protein, that permit dieters to enjoy the taste of hamburgers, hot dogs, fried chicken, chili, tacos, milkshakes, and cocktails. By combining the most nutrition for the least calories with taste satisfaction and fun, the Ultimate Ratio offers advantages that no other single eating plan can provide. These advantages give overfat and obese dieters the greatest chance at achieving lifetime fat loss.

Protein seems to play an important role in the Ultimate Ratio plan, yet you criticize diet book authors who promote eating lots of protein. How do you justify this?

Protein is an essential nutrient that we must eat every day, and accordingly, the Ultimate Ratio contains high-quality protein derived from the world's healthiest foods in scientifically justifiable amounts. But the Ultimate Ratio is *not* a high-protein eating plan. High-protein diets (which are by their very nature also low in carbohydrates and high in fat) can wreak biochemical havoc in the body by causing dehydration (which cripples endurance and athletic performance and leads to the loss of such vital minerals as calcium and potassium in urine), constipation (due to insufficient fiber intake), bad breath (due to ketosis), dizziness (due to low blood pressure), and fatigue (caused by insufficient intake of carbohydrates). Since there is scant published scientific evidence that high-protein/low-carbohydrate diets promote fitness, health, and well-being and plenty of evidence to show that these diets can lead people to disease, I suspect that most protein-pushing diet book authors devised their diets first on speculation and only then rounded up whatever "evidence" they could find to support them.

That is precisely the opposite of what they should have done and the result is shoddy science. Most credible scientists reject the health and fitness claims made by these protein-pushing authors. But even those who don't should realize that their method—forming conclusions based on personal taste, speculation, and prejudice, and then rustling up support for them—invariably produces questionable results.

Why do you think high-protein/high-fat diet books have become so popular today? I've seen the same types of diets in various books over the last few decades, but they've always been scientifically discredited. What has changed?

The diets remain the same. What has changed is the level of frustration people feel after attempting to lose weight and failing repeatedly. Frustrated and disappointed dieters are vulnerable to promises of easy weight loss. The architects of high-protein/high-fat diets seduce their readers using the same propaganda technique favored by despots, bigots, and dictators: They rally support against a scapegoat. This is a time-honored technique that helps shift blame away from the true causes of people's failures and frustrations and toward an innocent victim. The scapegoat, in this case, is carbohydrates. They tell readers that it's not their fault that they are fat or obese. They blame it all on carbohydrates. If only this were true! Of course, it isn't, but that simple message is one that many frustrated dieters find easy to swallow.

I've seen stories on TV tabloid shows and in supermarket tabloids about people who have lost weight on popular high-protein/high-fat diets. How can you dispute the success of these weight-loss diets?

I've never counseled a single obese individual (someone with a BMI greater than 30) who ever stayed slender (achieving a BMI between 17 and 22) on a high-protein/high-fat (HPHF) diet. If you have been observant, you have probably noticed that most dieters who have been interviewed on TV tabloid shows and in the press remain overfat (as do most of the authors of HPHF diet books) despite their "success" on an HPHF diet. Sadly, few of them stand a chance of ever becoming permanently slender. In fact, studies show they actually stand a much greater chance of eventually gaining all the lost weight back, plus more. There's a good reason for that. An HPHF diet creates a metabolic *imbalance* in the body called ketosis. A person in ketosis loses his or her appetite and begins eating fewer calories—so far, so good. Unfortunately, there's no such thing as a free lunch. Eventually, the body rebels against this chemical imbalance because all of us have a genetically programmed "carbohydrate instinct" hard-wired into our genes. They begin craving and eating carbohydrates—slowly at first. Most people justify these forbidden carbohydrate indulgences by telling themselves, "I'm on a *modified* version of the (fill in the name of your favorite HPHF diet)." But once they modify an HPHF diet by consuming more carbohydrate-rich foods, the fat-loss game is over. Ketosis comes to a screeching halt, and their appetite returns with a vengeance. Only now they have developed a taste for rich and fatty foods and cannot easily return to a healthy way of eating. That's why you will most likely never meet a formerly obese, slender person who reached and maintained their healthy weight on an HPHF diet.

The Ultimate Ratio emphasizes eating protein-dense and carbohydrate-rich foods within the same meal. A best-selling diet book I read claims that combining carbohydrates with proteins in the same meal will make me fat. Is this true?

A popular fad diet book written not by a nutritionist but by a TV star advises readers that if they eat fruit, they should do so four hours before or after they eat anything else. This diet limits carbohydrate consumption to 10 grams a day for the first two weeks, and then up to 20 grams a day thereafter. It also promotes the consumption of eggs, red meats, cheese, cream cheese, and pork rinds, and offers a limited list of vegetables. It discourages consumption of such foods as potatoes, pasta, bread, and rice. The book's author resurrects an erroneous theory of food combining which holds that eating certain combinations of nutrients, such as proteins and carbohydrates in the same meal, causes a variety of digestive and health problems because these nutrients require different enzymes for their digestion. Other proponents of this food-combining theory claim that eating a protein-dense food such as meat with a high-carbohydrate food such as a baked potato will interfere with digestion, which will then cause the undigested food to ferment and putrefy, spending up to two years in the colon! This is science fiction. Digestion actually begins in the mouth, continuing in the stomach and in the small intestine. Pancreatic fluid is secreted into the small intestine and contains enzymes that digest proteins, carbohydrates, and fats. Humans evolved on a diet of mixed foods, and no human population has ever subsisted on eating single foods at a time. Diet book authors who espouse this food-combining theory claim that when you don't digest foods properly, you get fat. Exactly the opposite happens. If you don't completely digest foods, you absorb *fewer* calories and you lose weight.

How did you discover the Mediterrasian Diet?

In the late 1970s, I discovered that a very low-fat vegetarian diet (10 percent fat) could reverse the buildup of arterial plaque in patients I counseled at my nutrition clinic. In 1980, I tried to get the Department of Cardiology at a major medical center in Miami, Florida, to implement and test my diet in their patients with heart disease. These cardiologists emphatically denied that it was possible to reverse arterial plaque buildup with diet. Sadly, they refused to allow their cardiac patients to follow such a diet. Of course, they were eventually proven to be wrong, and I often wonder how many of their patients' lives could have been saved had they been allowed to participate in the proposed study. This disappointment plus the fact that most of my clients had trouble sticking to such a strict diet while trying to maintain a normal social life, which included dining out and going to parties and affairs, led me to examine more "socially friendly" eating plans that might work just as well. When I studied the diets of other cultures in which cardiovascular disease was rare, I discovered that certain foods in the diets of Mediterranean peasants and native Japanese seemed to provide powerful protection against heart disease, obesity, and other serious health problems yet were still delicious and satisfying. I isolated these foods, analyzed their nutritional content, investigated the biochemical effects of their respective nutrients, and devised a delicious way of eating that combined the healthiest and most slimming foods of the Mediterranean and Asian diets. These foods include soy foods and beverages (e.g., "hamburgers," "hot dogs," and "milkshakes" made from soy protein), tomato sauces, fruits, seafood, vegetables, chocolate, coffee, cocoa, wine, tea, rice, pasta, potatoes, and oatmeal. Within those general categories, I was able to further refine my recommendations to emphasize the most nutritious foods. For example, among fruits, blueberries, strawberries, and citrus fruits provide the most powerful antioxidant activity. Such seafood as salmon, mackerel, and tuna contains friendly fats that help fight heart disease and cancer. Tomato sauces, crucifers (e.g., broccoli and cabbage), soybeans and other legumes provide peak performance nutrients for eat-to-winners. And olive oil, forbidden on a very low-fat diet (10 percent fat), can be used as a tasty, disease-fighting ingredient to make recipes more flavorful and satisfying. This *Mediterrasian Diet* (a term I coined to describe the unique dietary foundation of the Ultimate Ratio plan) provides the most powerful combination of foods and beverages of any diet I have ever examined. A recent study of 605 heart disease patients found that those following a Mediterranean-type diet rich in legumes, seafood, fresh fruits, vegetables, and olive oil cut their risk of death by 56 percent compared to patients who ate an ordinary American diet. People in the study also reduced their risk of developing cancer by 61 percent. Researchers noted that people with heart disease in the study found that a Mediterranean-type diet proved to be a tastier alternative to the typical low-fat diet (10 percent fat) often prescribed by nutritionists. The Ultimate Ratio plan offers a delicious alternative to those people who find a very low-fat diet difficult or impossible to follow.

What dietary supplements do you take?

My entire dietary supplement regimen consists of three recipes that I have given you in this book: I use the **Phyto Mary Cocktail** recipe every morning. This supplies a complete multi-vitamin mineral formulation with a powerful profile of disease-fighting phytonutrients. It doesn't get any better than this. I drink the **Purple Cow Shake** recipe for breakfast or lunch or as an afternoon snack. This recipe contains soy isoflavones, high-quality protein, and antioxidants, which help repair exercise-induced muscle damage and rebuild muscle tissue as well as protect against cancer, heart disease, diabetes, and osteoporosis. When I need additional mental energy, focus, and concentration, I use the **Orange Genius Shake.** This is an amazing drink that keeps me alert and focused all day. In fact, I was able to research long hours and write this book thanks to the mental fitness nutrients in the **Orange Genius.** My athletic clients love the increased performance they enjoy from using it and have set several world records thanks to its ability to enhance the mind-body connection. Sometimes I use the **Orange Genius** recipe (p. 166) for a morning pick-me-up in place of coffee. These three recipes provide complete supplemental nutrition. I avoid nutritional supplements that contain iron because many of the foods in our food supply are already iron-fortified and because I get my iron from such foods as legumes and other vegetables. It's easy to consume too much iron, and excess iron can injure blood vessels and cause heart disease, cancer, and liver and kidney damage. Many physicians routinely prescribe iron supplements to their patients without recognizing these consequences. Most healthy people who follow the Ultimate Ratio can get all the iron they need from vegetables, soy foods, and whole grains.

Why are functional foods and beverages so important on the Ultimate Ratio Plan?

If you want to lose excess body fat and keep it off permanently, functional foods and drinks provide a revolutionary means to help you achieve your goal. That's because they provide the most nutrition for the least calories. They also supplant the calorically dense and unhealthy foods in our diet, such as fried foods and fast foods. The recommended functional foods and drinks on the Ultimate Ratio plan make it easy for dieters to obtain enough vitamins, minerals, and phytonutrients during periods of caloric restriction. Old-school dietitians and nutritionists still argue that we can get all the nutrients we need from foods. That's assuming that people will chose healthy, nutrient-dense foods, which is rarely the case. In fact, 25 percent of the vegetables consumed in the United States are French fries—America's favorite vegetable! If you want to safeguard against the diseases of aging (such as cancer, heart disease, hypertension, arthritis, senility, and loss of vision and hearing), you will most likely benefit from using functional foods and drinks. Functional foods and drinks are not meant to replace the nutrients in foods, but merely to supplement them. That's why they are called dietary supplements. *Caution: Always check with a physician before taking dietary supplements, including those mentioned in this book.*

Are any of the so-called metabolism booster dietary supplements safe and effective?

A safe and effective weight-loss pill that melts away excess body fat would be the answer to every dieter's prayers. Could a simple herb or food supplement succeed where prescription diet pills have failed? That's the premise and the promise of a new generation of dietary supplements that curb appetite and speed up fat burning in the body.

Published studies on long-term weight loss reveal that most people rarely succeed on their own. Many people require a motivational boost to help them jump-start a new diet. Despite the dangers associated with using appetite suppressants and metabolism boosters, many dieters seem willing to face such side effects as dizziness, edginess, and insomnia, or worse if it means they can slip into slender-cut fashions instead of struggling to fit into plus-sizes.

Ever since July 1998, when the FDA ordered manufacturers of the two very popular weight-loss drugs—fenfluramine and phentermine (collectively known as "fen-phen")—to remove them from the market, physicians and their overweight patients have been scrambling to find safe and effective replacements. The diet-pill recall came after researchers at the Mayo Clinic linked fenfluramine to heart-valve abnormalities in two dozen patients. Seriously obese patients who had lost as much as 100 pounds using the drugs were left without the pharmacological crutch they desperately needed to help them lose weight and keep it off.

Although most health experts agree that the questions surrounding fen-phen were serious enough to warrant drastic action, no one really knows whether the drugs have actually harmed people. Ironically, the withdrawal of these effective weight-loss drugs from the market could cause harm as well as good. Many obesity specialists warn that the loss of these drugs could set back obesity treatment many years.

Recently, dietary supplement companies have offered fat-loss products that promise to curb appetite and boost thermogenesis (fat burning). Scientific studies published in peer-reviewed science journals suggest that these products, when used as directed by healthy adults, appear to be safe and effective—at least in the short run. No long-term studies exist to assure dieters that they won't suffer health consequences with long-term use. But these products actually work, and that alone may be enough to entice physicians and frustrated dieters—especially those who face such obesity-related health problems as heart disease, adult-onset diabetes, osteoarthritis, hypertension, and cancer—to use them.

Only two effective metabolism boosters are found in over-the-counter (OTC) dietary supplements. Ephedrine is the active ingredient in the most popular fat-loss products. Ephedrine is derived from the herb ephedra, which has been used in Chinese medicine for thousands of years. A synthetic version of the compound has been added to nonprescription cold and asthma medications since the 1920s. Studies show that ephedrine curbs appetite, boosts metabolism, improves concentration, and most important, burns fat. Some users claim that the herb enhances sexual performance. A small number of published scientific studies suggest that the herb can be used for up to six months to achieve significant body fat loss. Currently, ephedra can be found in more than 200 diet supplements (capsules, pills, powders, drinks, and diet candy bars) for sale in health food stores and on the Internet. The other effective fat-burning compound is citrus aurantium (also known as synephrine). To date, only one dietary supplement manufacturer (Twin Laboratories) has developed a citrus aurantium–based fat-burning formula. It is sold in capsules, drinks, and candy bars called Metabolift. Metabolift products are available in two formulations: those that contain ephedra and those that contain synephrine.

One recently published scientific study revealed that the Metabolift formula containing citrus aurantium was found to be effective in promoting fat loss when used with mild caloric restriction and regular, moderate exercise. The reported success of Metabolift bodes well for dieters who have been starved for such news since the withdrawal of fen-phen from the marketplace. Because citrus aurantium–based supplements cause weight loss similar to that of the banned prescription diet pills, Pondamin (fenfluramine) and Redux (dexfenfluramine), many dieters have switched to these supplements to jump-start their fat-loss plans and keep motivation high when they need it the most—during the first weeks or months of their new diet.

Scientists are convinced that dietary supplements containing ephedra (often found in combination with caffeine to prolong its fat-burning effect) and citrus aurantium significantly stoke the body's fat-burning furnace. What remains in question is their safety. The FDA has received hundreds of calls about side effects reportedly linked to ephedra use. Some of these, which included dizziness, gastrointestinal distress, nervousness, insomnia, and even psychosis and death, have prompted the FDA to scrutinize the safety of ephedra. Even though millions of American dieters already use the herb with apparent success (judging from the astronomical sales of ephedra-containing products), the FDA remains unconvinced about the herb's safety. Even if ephedra is eventually proven to be safe when used as directed and for limited periods of time, many people should not use the herb, including those with heart disease, hypertension, diabetes, thyroid disease, kidney and liver disease, and those who are pregnant or breast-feeding. People with mental problems or those sensitive to ephedra and/or caffeine should not use these substances. People who believe that if "a little is good, more is better" should also avoid using ephedra and other metabolism boosters because that is definitely *not* the case with these powerful substances. Even healthy adults probably should not use ephedra or any other metabolism booster indefinitely. *Anyone who contemplates using products that curb appetite or speed up the body's metabolic rate should check with a physician before doing so.*

Even though I have used metabolism boosters in my nutritional practice with success, I do not endorse their indiscriminant use. These products do not supplant a healthy low-calorie diet and exercise program, but they do help obese dieters at risk of serious health problems curb their appetite and burn more body fat than they would using diet and exercise alone. It is important to recognize that the use of these and similar weight-loss products generally carry some health risks. I recommend that anyone who wants to use a metabolism booster that contains ephedra or any other fat-burning nutrient do so only under a physician's guidance. These potentially dangerous supplements may help jump-start your fat loss initially, but only a healthy diet and exercise plan will lead to lifetime slenderness.

Andre Agassi used a popular fat-burning supplement to help him shed excess body fat and develop the highly coveted "ripped" look defined by good muscle tone and low levels of subcutaneous fat. If you want to emulate Andre, first ask your doctor if these products are right for you. An ounce of prevention is worth a pound (or twenty or thirty pounds) of cure.

The height and weight charts I see in books and magazines indicate that I don't need to lose weight. I'm a forty-year-old female. My height is five feet six inches, and I weigh 140 pounds. Are these charts accurate?

For centuries the definition of fatness has been more a matter of taste than a science. In centuries past, carrying an extra 20 or 30 or 40 pounds signified wealth and a high social standing. More recently, insurance companies set the standards in the United States for healthy height and weight. Their definitions of fatness and obesity were far too generous. Even the government's guidelines, until quite recently, allowed too much weight for a given height. If you are an office worker who plays tennis on the weekends, you are most likely overfat at 140 pounds. On the other hand, a professional female athlete of your height who has relatively large amounts of muscle tissue would probably not be overfat at 140 pounds. If you find height and weight charts confusing, you can use the "eyeball test" instead. Look at your unclothed body in a full-length mirror (preferably a three-way mirror that affords you a front and rear view). Do not focus only on your face and block out the rest of your body (many overfat people tend to do this whenever they see their own reflection). You will instantly know if you are overfat.

I eat very little, yet I still gain weight. Is there something wrong with my metabolism?

Most likely the fault lies with your memory and not your metabolic rate. Published studies reveal that most people have a selective memory about what they consume over time. These studies show that people tend to underestimate their food intake when researchers ask them to recall what they eat over the course of a week or even several days. If you are gaining weight, you are eating too much fat (the only nutrient that will add fat to your body) and too many calories, which will prevent your body from releasing and burning its stored fat. You may also not be getting enough exercise to partially empty your glycogen tank each day.

Even though I'm fat, I am comfortable with my body so why should I lose weight?

In over twenty years of counseling overfat people, I have never met a single soul who—in a totally honest moment—did not confess to being unhappy about being overfat. It's understandable when someone who has failed repeatedly to lose fat or to keep lost fat from returning embraces this philosophy of acceptance. In truth, it is a rare person who is comfortable with being fat or obese. Do not confuse complacency with comfort. The two are quite different.

Even though I'm fat, my spouse never complains. So why should I worry about losing weight?

As many times as I've heard that sentence uttered by my clients (and it has been far too many times to count over the years), I seem to remember also hearing their spouse complain to me privately that they should lose weight. More than 50 percent of marriages end in divorce. I would guess that a significant number of failed marriages are due—directly or indirectly—to the fact that one of the spouses became fat or obese while the other spouse did not. A physically unappealing spouse can unwittingly drive his or her mate into an affair simply because they have "let themselves go." It's a shame, but it happens many times every day the world over.

People shouldn't judge me or belittle me because I'm fat. It's more important what's on the inside than the outside. I think I'm a nice person with many wonderful attributes, so why should I care about losing weight?

This is a variation of the old saying, "Don't judge a book by its cover." While this is a wonderful sentiment and no one should ever be judged or discriminated against for being overfat or obese, it is no surprise that many people find the sight of fat unappealing. You may be the smartest, friendliest, and kindest human being ever to walk the earth, but published studies reveal that you *will* be discriminated against if you are overfat or obese. We can only speculate as to why people find the sight of excess body fat unappealing, but the fact is that overfat people are often treated as second-class citizens in school, at the office, and perhaps even in their own homes. You may be a best-selling book on the inside, but many people will never look beneath your cover because of your size. Study after study reveals that in our society, being overfat or obese *does* matter.

I've read that losing weight won't make me live any longer. Is that true?

It is quite difficult to prove beyond a shadow of a doubt that being fat kills people early, but what is clear is that overfat and obese people suffer a higher risk of several life-threatening conditions, including cardiovascular diseases, high blood pressure, Type II diabetes, several types of cancer, and numerous other medical conditions. Studies have shown that losing as little as 5 percent to 10 percent of one's body fat can reduce the risk of those conditions. When someone gains weight, the risk rises. Weight stability, compared with weight gain, will reduce mortality risk, so even if you can't lose weight, you shouldn't gain any more.

I've read that scientists have discovered that eating eggs won't raise your blood cholesterol level. Do I really need to avoid eating cholesterol-rich egg yolks, red meats, and butter as you recommend?

After seeing media stories about recent studies that exonerate eggs from raising blood cholesterol levels, you might have thought: "I've been avoiding eggs all these years for no good reason. I think I'll start enjoying a three-egg omelet for breakfast." Here's the scoop on eggs: Eating eggs won't significantly raise the blood cholesterol level in most people who eat a typical Western diet because their blood is already fairly saturated with cholesterol. Published studies reveal that whenever people with blood cholesterol levels below 150 milligrams (the upper limit for a healthy blood cholesterol level) start eating eggs, their blood cholesterol soars and reaches the level found in most ordinary Americans—who die of heart disease in epidemic numbers. People with long-standing blood cholesterol levels below 150 milligrams rarely have heart attacks. In fact, researchers involved with the famous Framingham Heart Study (an ongoing study which was begun in 1948) found that people in the study with blood cholesterol levels below 150 milligrams did not develop heart disease. But they did find plenty of people who suffered heart attacks with blood cholesterol levels between 200 and 260 milligrams—the same range of values typically found in people who eat eggs, red meats, poultry, and cheese and other high-fat dairy products. There are many dietary factors that raise blood cholesterol levels, including saturated fats (found mainly in animal foods), trans-fatty acids (found in many commercially prepared baked goods), sugar, psychological stress, and eating too many calories from all foods. The typical daily cholesterol intake for most adults is 350 to 400 milligrams. On the Ultimate Ratio, my blood cholesterol number usually hovers around 140 milligrams. As an experiment, I once switched to a high-protein/high-fat diet for sixteen weeks. My blood cholesterol jumped eighty points to 220 milligrams—the value found among the majority of Americans who have heart disease. When I returned to the Ultimate Ratio plan, my cholesterol dropped to 144 milligrams in just four weeks. I recommend consuming, on average, no more than 700 milligrams of cholesterol each week. You don't have to completely avoid eating eggs (or any other food) on the Ultimate Ratio, but you should know that eating them does contribute to raising your blood cholesterol level if it is low (below 150 milligrams) and keeping it elevated if it is already moderate to high (200 to 260 milligrams).

The Ultimate Ratio emphasizes vegetables as its foundation and soy foods as an important protein source, yet the USDA's Food Guide Pyramid emphasizes grains and cereals as its foundation and doesn't even mention soy foods. Who is correct?

The USDA's Food Guide Pyramid appears to be a sellout to the dairy, egg, and meat lobbies. When the USDA first released its Food Guide Pyramid, the recommended portions of beef and dairy products were relatively small. But food industry lobbyists forced the USDA to revise its Food Guide Pyramid. After spending an additional year and one million dollars of taxpayer money, the USDA issued a new Food Guide Pyramid—this time, with more generous portions of meat and dairy products nearly identical to those it had recommended back in the 1950s. The Ultimate Ratio emphasizes vegetables as a primary carbohydrate source for fat loss instead of grains and cereals because vegetables contain far more vitamins, minerals, and phytonutrients per calorie than do grains and cereals. It's easier to lose fat and maintain fat loss by consuming a diet based on vegetables and low-fat soy foods. Unlike the USDA Pyramid, the Ultimate Ratio limits red meats, egg yolks, and full-fat dairy products because they are too high in fat, cholesterol, and calories for optimal health and permanent fat loss.

Some of the foods and products you recommend are expensive. Fresh salmon, functional beverages, and such functional foods as soy-based bacon, sausage, hot dogs, and hamburger seem pricey when compared to many other foods. Can I really afford to eat according to the Ultimate Ratio?

In my opinion, you can't afford to exclude these healthy foods from your diet. A few extra dollars spent at the supermarket can mean the difference between optimal health and disease. Salmon, soy drink mixes, and soy meat replacers all contain powerful vitamins, minerals, and natural disease-fighting chemicals that can help you achieve lifetime slenderness and excellent health. Are they worth the money? They are worth it if you value looking good, feeling good, and achieving better health.

You claim that the body can only store dietary fat directly as body fat. Does that mean I will lose weight simply by avoiding all fats and eating all the potatoes, pasta, rice, fruits, and vegetables I care to eat?

You should not avoid all fats, nor should you gorge on any one type of food. Some fats are healthy and are essential to achieving optimal health. Fats found in such foods as soy foods, salmon, tuna, and olive oil are heart-friendly, which means they will not raise your blood cholesterol level. When you want to lose weight or maintain your weight loss, you should limit your intake of all fats to the levels I recommend in this book. The body stores almost all the fats in the foods you eat (called triglycerides) directly as body fat after first breaking them down in the digestive tract and then reassembling them to again form triglycerides in the liver and transporting them in the bloodstream to fat cells. Proteins and carbohydrates are not stored directly as fat. The body uses proteins for growth, repair, and maintenance, and to synthesize chemicals that help the body function normally. It uses carbohydrates mainly as fuel and stores the excess you eat in the liver and muscles as glycogen. Although your body can manufacture its own fat from all foods and alcohol under certain conditions, dietary fat is really the only nutrient that adds fat directly to your body.

You recommend oatmeal over all popular dry fat-free breakfast cereals. I thought these breakfast cereals were good for me. Please explain your preference for oatmeal.

Many fat-free, dry breakfast cereals are loaded with sugar and calories. Dry cereals are so calorically dense that ounce for ounce they supply over three times the calories of cooked oatmeal. Oatmeal contains healthy phytonutrients, so it is clearly a wiser choice for anyone who wants to lose fat while enjoying cereal for breakfast.

How many calories should I consume each day to lose excess body fat?

This is a very individual question, but I can give you some rough guidelines. A sedentary woman who is five feet, four inches tall and weighs 140 pounds might maintain her body weight while consuming just 1,400 calories each day. A sedentary man who is five feet, nine inches tall and weighs 175 pounds could maintain his body weight while eating just 1,700 calories a day. Surprisingly, these amounts are less than the caloric intakes for weight maintenance recommended by most health organizations. Many people may find it difficult to limit their calorie intake to these levels because so many of the foods served in restaurants and sold in supermarkets are calorically dense. Of course, restaurant portions have also increased during the last decade, making it even more difficult to keep from gaining weight. Fortunately, the Ultimate Ratio recommended foods are rich in flavor, provide maximum satiety, and are low in calories. This allows you to enjoy a larger volume of tasty foods (even fast food "burgers," "shakes," "fried chicken," and "hot dogs") while consuming a relatively low-calorie diet. Most women and men who are physically active will consume approximately 1,200 to 1,400 calories a day, respectively, on the Ultimate Ratio fat-loss plan when they want to lose excess body fat. According to my research, once you meet your daily need for protein, vitamins, and minerals (easily achieved on as little as 1,000 to 1,200 calories when you follow the Ultimate Ratio plan), the fewer calories you consume, the healthier you will be. This is consistent with the anti-aging theory known as CRAN (**c**aloric **r**estriction with **a**dequate **n**utrition), a diet strategy that has already been shown to exert powerful life-extending effects in laboratory animals. It has yet to be conclusively shown that CRAN will starve off the diseases of aging in humans, but thus far there is every indication that it will work in humans as well as it does in laboratory animals. Current research projects investigating CRAN in humans will one day establish whether this is true. Once you reach your target weight, you can slowly adjust your caloric intake upward using the Ultimate Ratio weight-maintenance plan to stabilize your new body weight.

Why hasn't anyone ever explained how important controlling the body's glycogen level is to achieving permanent fat loss?

Actually, a number of researchers who publish articles in scientific journals have theorized that controlling the body's glycogen level is the key to achieving lifetime slimness. Critics counter that no one has proven conclusively that glycogen plays a role in controlling appetite and body fat levels, and they are correct for the moment. But a growing body of research suggests that when you consume a diet similar to the Ultimate Ratio and exercise regularly, your body's glycogen levels help control how full you feel (satiety) and whether or not you will burn excess body fat for fuel. Based on my research, I am convinced that regulating the body's glycogen level does indeed lead to permanent fat loss. I used to be overweight, but I've been able to stay very slender, fit, and healthy for the last twenty-eight years by controlling my body's glycogen stores with the Ultimate Ratio plan.

Are all carbohydrates nutritionally equivalent? Do some carbohydrate foods have more calories than others? Are some healthier than others?

Carbohydrates supply about 4 calories per gram. There are two basic types of carbohydrates—simple and complex. Simple carbohydrates are found in table sugar, honey, syrup, and molasses. Complex carbohydrates are found in such foods as potatoes, rice, pasta, fruits, and legumes. Most natural foods, particularly fruits, contain a mixture of simple and complex carbohydrates. Such minimally processed complex carbohydrate foods as brown rice and oatmeal contain various types of fiber, which is noncaloric and aids in digestion and elimination. In general, simple carbohydrates are digested more rapidly than complex carbohydrates and released into the bloodstream faster. Recent studies have linked a high intake of simple carbohydrates to such diseases as type II diabetes and cardiovascular disease. On average, American men and women eat their weight in sugar each year (about 160 pounds and 130 pounds, respectively). This is twice the amount recommended by many health experts and more than you would obtain by following the Ultimate Ratio plan. The ordinary American diet contains about 28 percent of its total calories as added sugar. The Ultimate Ratio provides about 10 percent of daily calories from added sugar.

I tried a low-fat/high-carbohydrate diet and gained weight, so why should I continue eating potatoes and other high-carbohydrate foods as you recommend?

Studies have shown that the majority of people who believe they've followed a low-fat/high-carbohydrate (LFHC) diet never even got close! Many people used the LFHC diet as a license to gorge on sugar and starches. Wolfing down an entire bag of fat-free cookies does not qualify as being on an LFHC diet. Deceptive packaging information and ignorance about food composition led many people to eat more fat and calories than they had previously eaten, causing many to gain weight while mistakenly believing they were eating less fat than before. In fact, they wound up eating more fat and more calories, except this time, the extra calories and extra fat came from such high-carbohydrate foods (loaded with hidden fat) as muffins, bagels, sugar-free baked goods, and air-popped popcorn. Here are just a few examples: Many people think of air-popped popcorn as "fantasy" food—meaning that it contains just hot air and virtually no calories. In fact, some brands of air-popped popcorn are sprayed with fat *after* popping. One popular brand of air-popped popcorn contains 170 calories and 11 fat grams per ounce. You'd actually consume fewer calories by snacking on regular potato chips instead (150 calories, 10 grams of fat per ounce). No-fat salad dressing is no caloric bargain either. A 4-ounce fat-free muffin sold in bake shops and grocery stores sounds like a good deal at 130 calories. If you read the fine print on the nutrition label, you'll discover that this value is for half the muffin. How many people do you know who eat just half a muffin? One bagel can contain 10 grams of fat, depending on how it was made, and 400 to 600 calories, depending on its size. Bagel chips can have up to six fat grams per serving. A number of popular fat-free salad dressings contain 60 calories per serving. Many high-carb foods contain plenty of calories, sugar, and lots of hidden fat. So don't delude yourself into thinking you are eating an LFHC diet if you eat these foods. The healthiest and most slimming LFHC foods are vegetables (including potatoes) and fruits. These are the most natural and least processed high-carbohydrate foods, and they are the ones that will not add fat to your body.

I've read that genetics plays a larger role than diet does in making people fat. Is that true?

Some genes can slow metabolism making it difficult to keep from gaining and re-gaining weight. But these genes are responsible for only a small percentage of people who are overfat and obese. Genetics only contributes to the propensity toward becoming obese. It does *not* doom people to obesity. Although a person's genes are partly responsible for obesity, their degree of fatness is largely determined by diet and lifestyle. Genes cannot explain the steep increase in weight gain among children and adults during the past twenty years because it takes tens of thousands of years for genes to evolve. Some minority groups, including African Americans, Hispanics, Native Americans and Pacific Islanders, are far more likely to be overweight than whites. But regardless of your genetic lineage, the Ultimate Ratio plan can help you achieve permanent fat loss because *no one* is impervious to the slimming effects of this eating plan and exercise. On the Ultimate Ratio plan, people can expect to lose excess body fat and keep it off for life—even those with a sluggish metabolic rate.

I see reports in the media almost daily about science and health. Are these reports usually accurate?

Newspapers, tabloids, and network and cable TV news shows tend to sensationalize new diet and health discoveries. Their reports are often superficial or incomplete because of time constraints or available space. They also want to grab and hold your attention, and so they tend to sensationalize science and health stories. Here are two examples of media health stories that alarmed the public but turned out to be much ado about nothing. Once you examine the facts, these stories seem far less sensational and important than as portrayed in the media.

1. The courts held the Dow Corning Company liable for the health problems of thousands of American women who received the company's breast implants. A jury ordered Dow Corning to pay out an enormous cash settlement to these women to compensate for their medical bills and suffering. In the Dow-Corning case, hundreds of women who had silicon breast implants made by the company were recruited to join a lawsuit against the corporation via attorneys' ads in the print media. The ads listed a constellation of symptoms connected to impaired immune system functions that were allegedly caused by the implants. The attorneys presented individuals' medical case histories and medical experts to convince the jury that implants caused immune system disorders in the plaintiffs. The jury believed them. Shortly after this landmark decision, the prestigious *New England Journal of Medi-*

cine published results of a scientific research trial involving thousands of women that found no connection whatsoever between immune system disorders and silicon breast implants. Subsequent studies have confirmed this original report. A small percentage of women in the United States had silicon breast implants, and a small percentage of women in the United States have immune system problems or disorders. What the jury never realized is that, by chance, there is some overlap of these populations and that there was no connection between silicon breast implants and immune disorders other than an accidental causal connection.

2. In recent years there has been a huge increase in the number of media stories about people who claim they were kidnapped by alien creatures from outer space, subjected to medical experiments, and then released again. A Roper Poll conducted in 1992 indicated that nearly four million Americans believe they have been abducted by aliens. I'm sure many people watching TV reportage of these *X-File*–like phenomena believe they have a degree of merit. The media tend to sensationalize such events in a way that doesn't dismiss them as flights of fancy or artifacts of the imagination. You might even believe that aliens are abducting *homo sapiens* and performing medical experiments on them and then releasing them, setting them down gently in their beds or in a field. (Of course, there will even be a few people reading this paragraph who will assume that I am an alien sent to divert suspicion from these abductions.) The majority of these cases are due to a medical phenomenon known as sleep paralysis, a condition that makes people feel as if they are transported out of their body. In medieval times, Europeans interpreted sleep paralysis as assaults or abductions by witches taking them off for a ride on a broomstick. People tend to draw upon the most plausible account in their cultural repertoire to explain their experience. Since goblins, trolls, and witches no longer constitute plausible interpretations of these hallucinations, people are more comfortable with the notion of aliens from outer space because it is more contemporary and (somewhat) more plausible to the modern mind. Thus, a flight on a witch's broomstick is replaced by a ride in an alien spacecraft where abductees are poked, probed, and prodded. The reports of alien abduction not due to sleep paralysis can be explained by false memories, daydreams, and fantasies, according to Leonard S. Newman, a psychologist at the University of Illinois at Chicago who has studied the alien abduction phenomenon.

Eat to Win for Permanent Fat Loss is your road map to health, fitness, and permanent fat loss. I hope the information I've presented will help you develop critical thinking so that you can better separate science fact from science fiction. *Eat to Win for Permanent Fat Loss* is based on the latest discoveries in nutritional science from thousands of peer-review published studies and my personal research and work with people from all walks of life and at all levels of fitness and health. I've devoted twenty-four years to the research and study of diet, health, and fitness to provide you with this cutting-edge nutritional knowledge. Now, it's *your* turn to do the work. If you are willing to follow the dietary principles I've given you, you will succeed where most others have failed.

I conclude this section with a final observation, alien abductions notwithstanding: The truth is out there.

RECIPES

FAVORITE MEALS
MADE BETTER

BLENDER DRINKS AND BEVERAGES

ENTRÉES, SNACKS, SIDES, AND DESSERTS

ULTIMATE RATIO RECIPE HINTS

Here are a few tips to make your cooking and shopping more convenient. Find out which supermarkets and natural-food stores near you stock the most frequently occurring ingredients in these recipes. If you have trouble finding any of these products, ask the store manager about ordering them. I've listed many of the food items by brand name in the recipes because they provide the best results. Reasonable substitutions are fine. You will find a complete list of food products, manufacturers, phone numbers, and web addresses in Appendix III, page 225.

Concerning Functional Drink Recipes

- Have on hand at least two ice cube trays with standard-size rectangular holes. You will find that cubes of juice and soy milk make the Ultimate Ratio Beverages extra delicious and rich in texture. (For reference: Every two frozen cubes of these beverages equal ⅓ cup liquid.) Once you and your family discover your favorite functional drink, you will know what cubes of frozen liquid to keep ready.
- Keep peeled and frozen bananas (tightly wrapped) on hand as well as bags of frozen berries.

  Prepare bananas for freezing as follows:
  1. Allow bananas to ripen fully.
  2. Peel and cut each banana into 4 pieces.
  3. Wrap all 4 pieces in one sheet of plastic.
  4. Repeat with each banana.
  5. Store the prepared bananas in a zippered freezer bag until ready to use.
- Always make new frozen cubes as you use them so you won't be disappointed when you go to the freezer with a craving for your favorite drink. It's easier to make blender drinks more quickly in the morning if you start them the night before. Measure out all the ingredients except the frozen ones (e.g., soy milk cubes, juice cubes, and frozen fruit) into the blender container, blend briefly, and store covered in the refrigerator overnight. In the morning, simply pulse the ingredients to remix them and add your frozen cubes and/or fruit and process until smooth. This way you are not forced to "think" before you've had one of these eye-opening smart drinks.

- Everyone who enjoys these shakes would do well to purchase a tall thermos cup. It will keep a shake frosty cold for hours.
- The blender drinks calling for Twinlab's Choline Cocktail contain caffeine. These are powerful "pick me up" beverages. Although they are fine for adults who are not caffeine sensitive, they should be avoided by individuals who have been advised by a physician to avoid caffeine and by children under twelve. I've placed a reminder to this effect at the bottom of each recipe containing Twinlab's Choline Cocktail.
- These Ultimate Ratio beverages not only leave out a lot of the "bad" stuff that traditional shakes and smoothies have, like fat-laden ice cream and sugary frozen yogurt, but also deliver supernutrition that heretofore could not be obtained in such a palatable form.

ABOUT YOUR NEW FOODS

These recipes are based on some of the most popular foods and fast foods in America. Most of them come together in minutes. Some take a little longer but can be prepared in stages. For example, you can make the Egg n' Muffins (page 180) up to several days ahead of time. They'll heat up in the microwave in seconds and taste freshly made. When preparing recipes calling for egg substitute, line the plate with wax paper or a paper towel before microwaving. Baked-on egg substitute can be difficult to remove.

Individual portions are no problem. Although the recipes usually serve four, many of the sandwiches are built one at a time in the directions. So it's easy to prepare one, two, or five servings depending on how many will be eating.

Whenever possible, serve a fresh vegetable along with lunch and dinner. Lightly steam a vegetable of choice and flavor with lemon juice if desired. Even though lunch and dinner recipes have such names as Big Max Burgers, "Meaty" Baked Ziti, and Lemon "Chicken," most of them have a vegetable as the main ingredient—the soybean. So eat up without pangs of guilt.

I hope you enjoy these new versions of our all-time favorite foods. They're almost as good tasting as the real thing and much, much better for you.

BLENDER DRINKS AND BEVERAGES

BREAKFAST AND MEAL REPLACEMENT SHAKES

○ Creamsicle Power Punch

Yield: one serving

1 cup Edensoy Original Soy Beverage
1 teaspoon Twinlab MaxiLIFE Soy Cocktail
1 teaspoon Twinlab Choline Cocktail
1 tablespoon Eagle Brand Fat Free Sweetened Condensed Milk (optional)
4 cubes frozen orange juice

In a blender combine the soy beverage, soy cocktail, choline cocktail, and optional condensed milk. Pulse to blend. Add the frozen cubes and process till smooth. Serve immediately.

NOTE: Choline Cocktail contains 200 mg caffeine per 4 tablespoons, the same amount found in a strongly brewed cup of coffee. This product should not be consumed by caffeine-sensitive individuals, young children, pregnant or breast-feeding

*women, people with any health condition or disease, including high blood pressure
or heart disease, or those wishing to eliminate caffeine from their diet.*

Nutritional Totals Per Serving

Kilocalorie breakdown: 26.8% protein, 52.5% carbohydrate, 20.6% fat
Calories: 279
Protein: 14.9 (g)
Carbohydrate: 29.2 (g)
Fat: 5.1 (g)
Cholesterol: 2 (mg)
Sodium: 158 (mg)

◯ Orange Genius

Yield: one serving

1 cup Edensoy Original Soy Beverage
1 teaspoon Twinlab Choline Cocktail
4 cubes frozen orange juice

In a blender combine the soy beverage and choline cocktail and pulse to
blend. Add the frozen cubes and process till smooth. Serve immediately.

Nutritional Totals Per Serving

Kilocalorie breakdown: 28.4% protein, 43.3% carbohydrate, 28.3% fat
Calories: 215
Protein: 11.3 (g)
Carbohydrate: 17.2 (g)
Fat: 5.0 (g)
Cholesterol: 0 (mg)
Sodium: 105 (mg)

NOTE: *Choline Cocktail contains 200 mg caffeine per 4 tablespoons, the same
amount found in a strongly brewed cup of coffee. This product should not be consumed by caffeine-sensitive individuals, young children, pregnant or breast-feeding
women, people with any health condition or disease, including high blood pressure
or heart disease, or those wishing to eliminate caffeine from their diet.*

○ Phyto Mary Cocktail

Yield: one serving

1¼ cups V-8 Spicy Hot Vegetable Juice

2 tablespoons Twinlab MaxiLIFE Phytonutrient Cocktail

2 to 4 tablespoons Minute Maid 100% Lemon Juice (or freshly squeezed)

Place all the ingredients into a cocktail shaker or blender and shake or pulse to blend. Pour into a tall glass over ice. Serve immediately with a celery stalk for garnish if desired.

To make a less spicy drink, use some plain V-8 in the recipe.

Nutritional Totals Per Serving

Kilocalorie breakdown: 6.7% protein, 93.3% carbohydrate, 0% fat

Calories: 87

Protein: 1.4 (g)

Carbohydrate: 18.8 (g)

Fat: 0 (g)

Cholesterol: 0 (mg)

Sodium: 975 (g)

○ Purple Cow

Yield: one serving

1 cup Ocean Spray *Lightstyle* Cran-Grape Juice Drink

1 teaspoon Twinlab MaxiLIFE Soy Cocktail

½ cup frozen blueberries

1 medium banana, peeled and frozen

In a blender combine the cran-grape juice and soy cocktail and pulse to blend. Add the frozen berries and banana and process till smooth. Serve immediately.

Nutritional Totals Per Serving

Kilocalorie breakdown: 6.3% protein, 90.7% carbohydrate, 0.7% fat

Calories: 210

Protein: 5.4 (g)

Carbohydrate: 47.0 (g)
Fat: 0.8 (g)
Cholesterol: 0 (mg)
Sodium: 143 (mg)

○ Thick Chocolate Malted

Yield: one serving

⅔ cup Westsoy 1% Lite Soy Beverage
1 teaspoon Twinlab MaxiLIFE Soy Cocktail
2 tablespoons Carnation Malted Milk
2 tablespoons Hershey's Lite Chocolate Syrup (Genuine Chocolate Flavor)
4 cubes frozen Westsoy 1% Lite Soy Beverage

In a blender combine the liquid soy beverage, soy cocktail, malted milk, and chocolate syrup. Pulse to blend. Add the frozen cubes and process till smooth. Serve immediately.

Nutrition Totals Per Serving

Kilocalorie breakdown: 13.7% protein, 70.8% carbohydrate, 15.5% fat
Calories: 252
Protein: 8.1 (g)
Carbohydrate: 42 (g)
Fat: 4.1 (g)
Cholesterol: 3 (mg)
Sodium: 285 (mg)

○ 7-Eleven Power Freeze

Yield: one serving

1 cup Ocean Spray *Lightstyle* Cran-Raspberry Juice Drink
1 cup frozen mixed berries
1 medium banana, peeled and frozen
1 teaspoon Twinlab Choline Cocktail

Put all the ingredients into a blender and process till smooth. Serve immediately. (The texture will be like a 7-Eleven Slurpee. It may help to use a long spoon when pouring the beverage from the blender into a tall cup or glass.)

Nutritional Totals Per Serving

Kilocalorie breakdown: 3.3% protein, 93.3 carbohydrate
Calories: 244
Protein: 1.8 (g)
Carbohydrate: 50.5 (g)
Fat: 0.8
Cholesterol: 0 (mg)
Sodium: 79 (mg)

○ Tropical Power Punch

Yield: one Serving

1 cup Ocean Spray *Lightstyle* Cran-Mango Juice Drink
1 teaspoon Twinlab MaxiLIFE Soy Cocktail
1 teaspoon Twinlab Choline Cocktail
1 tablespoon Eagle Brand Fat Free Sweetened Condensed Milk (optional)
4 cubes frozen pineapple juice

In a blender combine the cran-mango juice, soy cocktail, choline cocktail, and optional condensed milk, and pulse to blend. Add the frozen cubes and process till smooth. Serve immediately.

Nutritional Totals Per Serving

Kilocalorie breakdown: 8.0% protein, 91.5% carbohydrate, 0.5% fat
Calories: 189
Protein: 3.6 (g)
Carbohydrate: 41.1 (g)
Fat: 0.1 (g)
Cholesterol: 2 (mg)
Sodium: 135 (mg)

NOTE: Choline Cocktail contains 200 mg caffeine per 4 tablespoons, the same amount found in a strongly brewed cup of coffee. This product should not be consumed by caffeine-sensitive individuals, young children, pregnant or breast-feeding

women, people with any health condition or disease, including high blood pressure
or heart disease, or those wishing to eliminate caffeine from their diet.

COFFEE AND TEA DRINKS

○ Caffè Latte

Yield: one serving

1 cup Edensoy Original Soy Beverage
1½ ounces (1 shot) espresso (decaffeinated or regular)

Heat the soy beverage on the stovetop, in the microwave, or by steaming.
Make the espresso and add it to the hot soy milk. Stir. Serve immediately.

For an Iced Caffè Latte, pour the freshly made espresso over ice to cool,
add 1 cup cold soy beverage, and stir to blend. Add more ice, if desired, and
serve.

Instant espresso powder may be substituted for fresh espresso. Follow
label instructions.

Nutrition Totals Per Serving

Kilocalorie breakdown: 42.8% protein, 12.7% carbohydrate, 44.6% fat
Calories: 146
Protein: 10.8 (g)
Carbohydrate: 3.2 (g)
Fat: 5.0 (g)
Cholesterol: 0 (mg)
Sodium: 129 (mg)

○ Cappuccino Frappé

Yield: one serving

⅔ cup Westsoy 1% Lite Soy Beverage
1 teaspoon MaxiLIFE Soy Cocktail
2 heaping teaspoons Taster's Choice Instant Coffee (decaffeinated or regular)

2 tablespoons Eagle Brand Fat Free Sweetened Condensed Milk

4 cubes frozen Westsoy 1% Lite Soy Beverage

In a blender, combine the liquid soy beverage, soy cocktail, instant coffee, and condensed milk. Pulse to blend. Add the frozen cubes and process till smooth. Serve immediately.

Nutrition Totals Per Serving

Kilocalorie breakdown: 10.9% protein, 78.83% carbohydrate, 10.4% fat
Calories: 296
Protein: 8.0 (g)
Carbohydrate: 58 (g)
Fat: 3.4 (g)
Cholesterol: 3 (mg)
Sodium: 187 (mg)

○ Green Tea Granita (with Ginseng and Ginkgo)

Yield: one serving

1 cup Arizona Diet Green Tea with Ginseng

1 teaspoon Twinlab Choline Cocktail (contains ginkgo)

5 cubes frozen Arizona Diet Green Tea with Ginseng

In a blender, combine the liquid green tea and choline cocktail and pulse to blend. Add the frozen cubes and process until the beverage turns slushy. Serve immediately.

Nutrition Totals Per Serving

Kilocalorie breakdown: 0% protein, 0% carbohydrate, 0% fat
Calories: 12
Protein: 0 (g)
Carbohydrate: 0 (g)
Fat: 0 (g)
Cholesterol: 0 (mg)
Sodium: 27 (mg)

NOTE: *Choline Cocktail contains 200 mg caffeine per 4 tablespoons, the same amount found in a strongly brewed cup of coffee. This product should not be consumed by caffeine-sensitive individuals, young children, pregnant or breast-feeding women, people with any health condition or disease, including high blood pressure or heart disease, or those wishing to eliminate caffeine from their diet.*

◯ High Tea Slush

Yield: one serving

½ cup Edensoy Original Soy Beverage
1 teaspoon Twinlab Choline Cocktail
⅔ cup Arizona Diet Iced Tea
4 to 6 cubes frozen Arizona Diet Iced Tea

In a blender, combine the soy beverage, choline cocktail, and liquid tea. Pulse to blend. Add the frozen cubes and process till beverage turns slushy. Serve immediately.

Nutritional Totals Per Serving

Kilocalorie breakdown: 41.9% protein, 10.9% carbohydrate, 47.2% fat
Calories: 77
Protein: 5.0 (g)
Carbohydrate: 1.3 (g)
Fat: 2.5 (g)
Cholesterol: 0 (mg)
Sodium: 66 (mg)

NOTE: *Choline Cocktail contains 200 mg caffeine per 4 tablespoons, the same amount found in a strongly brewed cup of coffee. This product should not be consumed by caffeine-sensitive individuals, young children, pregnant or breast-feeding women, people with any health condition or disease, including high blood pressure or heart disease, or those wishing to eliminate caffeine from their diet.*

◯ Mocha Freeze

Yield: one serving

⅔ cup Westsoy 1% Lite Soy Beverage
1 teaspoon Twinlab MaxiLIFE Soy Cocktail
2 heaping teaspoons Taster's Choice Instant Coffee (decaffeinated or regular)

2 tablespoons Hershey's Lite Chocolate Syrup

4 cubes frozen Westsoy 1% Lite Soy Beverage

In a blender, combine the liquid soy beverage, soy cocktail, instant coffee, and chocolate syrup. Pulse to blend. Add the frozen cubes and process till smooth. Serve immediately.

Nutrition Totals Per Serving

Kilocalorie breakdown: 19.3% protein, 67.4% carbohydrate, 13.4% fat
Calories: 214
Protein: 9.4 (g)
Carbohydrate: 32.9 (g)
Fat: 2.9 (g)
Cholesterol: 0 (mg)
Sodium: 196 (mg)

COCKTAIL HOUR ALCOHOLIC BEVERAGES

○ Healthy Bloody Mary

Yield: one serving

1 cup V-8 Spicy Hot Vegetable Juice

2 tablespoons Twinlab MaxiLIFE Phytonutrient Cocktail

2 to 4 tablespoons Minute Maid 100% Pure Lemon Juice (or freshly squeezed)

1 to 2 ounces flavored vodka (pepper or citrus)

1 celery stalk (optional)

Place all ingredients but the celery stalk into a cocktail shaker or blender and shake or pulse to blend. Pour into a tall glass over ice and garnish with the celery stalk.

Nutrition Totals Per Serving

Kilocalorie breakdown: 22.4% protein, 77.6% carbohydrate, 0.0% fat
Calories: 175
Protein: 2.2 (g)
Carbohydrate: 7.6 (g)
Fat: 0.0 (g)
Cholesterol: 0.0 (mg)
Sodium: 680 (mg)

◯ Perfect Piña Colada

Yield: one serving

½ cup Edensoy Original Soy Beverage
1 teaspoon Twinlab MaxiLIFE Soy Cocktail
1 to 2 ounces light rum
1 tablespoon coconut flavoring
2 tablespoons Eagle Fat Free Sweetened Condensed Milk
6 cubes frozen pineapple juice
Maraschino cherry and fresh pineapple wedge (optional)

In a blender, combine the soy beverage and soy cocktail and pulse to blend. Add the remaining ingredients and process till smooth. Serve immediately, garnished with a maraschino cherry and fresh pineapple wedge if desired.

Kids can enjoy this drink without the rum.

Nutritional Totals Per Serving

Kilocalorie breakdown: 14.6% protein, 76.9% carbohydrate, 8.5% fat
Calories: 391
Protein: 10.1 (g)
Carbohydrate: 53.0 (g)
Fat: 3.0 (g)
Cholesterol: 3 (mg)
Sodium: 136 (mg)

◯ The Un-Screwdriver

Yield: one serving

1 cup orange juice
1 tablespoon Twinlab Choline Cocktail
1 tablespoon Twinlab MaxiLIFE Phytonutrient Cocktail
2 ounces citrus-flavored vodka

Combine all the ingredients in a cocktail shaker or blender and shake or pulse to blend. Pour into a glass over ice. Serve immediately.

Nutrition Totals Per Serving

Kilocalorie breakdown: 6.6% protein, 93.4% carbohydrate, 0% fat
Calories: 284
Protein: 2.0 (g)
Carbohydrate: 28.5 (g)
Fat: 0 (g)
Cholesterol: 0 (mg)
Sodium: 0 (mg)

NOTE: Choline Cocktail contains 200 mg caffeine per 4 tablespoons, the same amount found in a strongly brewed cup of coffee. This product should not be consumed by caffeine-sensitive individuals, young children, pregnant or breast-feeding women, people with any health condition or disease, including high blood pressure or heart disease, or those wishing to eliminate caffeine from their diet.

SNACK AND DESSERT DRINKS

○ Banana Euphoria

Yield: two servings

1 cup Edensoy Original Soy Beverage

1 teaspoon Twinlab MaxiLIFE Soy Cocktail

1 large or 1½ medium bananas, peeled and frozen

2 tablespoons Eagle Brand Fat Free Sweetened Condensed Milk

1 teaspoon banana flavoring (optional)

In a blender, combine the soy beverage and soy cocktail and pulse to blend. Add the remaining ingredients and process till smooth. Serve immediately.

Nutritional Totals Per Serving

Kilocalorie breakdown: 10.3% protein, 82.6% carbohydrate, 7.0% fat
Calories: 189
Protein: 4.9 (g)
Carbohydrate: 39.6 (g)
Fat: 1.5 (g)
Cholesterol: 1.5 (mg)
Sodium: 98 (mg)

○ Rich Hot Cocoa

Yield: one serving

1 8.5-ounce envelope Swiss Miss Hot Cocoa Mix (no sugar added)
1 cup reduced-fat soy beverage, like Westsoy 1% Lite (or ½ cup Edensoy Original Soy
    beverage and ½ cup water)
Ready Whip Fat Free Dairy Whipped Topping (optional)

Empty contents of the envelope into a cup. In a separate container, heat the
soy beverage (and water, if using) on the stove or in the microwave. Pour
the hot liquid over the cocoa powder. Stir. Serve immediately. Garnish with
the whipped topping, if desired.

Nutrition Totals Per Serving

Kilocalorie breakdown: 15.9% protein, 66.2% carbohydrate, 17.9% fat
Calories: 160
Protein: 6.0 (g)
Carbohydrate: 25 (g)
Fat: 3 (g)
Cholesterol: 0 (mg)
Sodium: 280 (mg)

○ Super Strawberry Shake

Yield: two servings

1 cup Edensoy Original Soy Beverage
1 teaspoon Twinlab MaxiLIFE Soy Cocktail
3 tablespoons Eagle Brand Fat Free Sweetened Condensed Milk
1 heaping cup frozen strawberries (unsweetened)

In a blender, combine the soy beverage, soy cocktail, and condensed milk.
Pulse to blend. Add the strawberries and process till smooth. Serve immediately.

Nutrition Totals Per Serving

Kilocalorie breakdown: 19.2% protein, 70.0% carbohydrate, 10.8% fat
Calories: 178
Protein: 8.6 (g)
Carbohydrate: 31.3 (g)
Fat: 2.4 (g)
Cholesterol: 3 (mg)
Sodium: 101 (mg)

ENTRÉES, SNACKS, SIDES, AND DESSERTS

BREAKFAST

○ Awesome Oatmeal

Yield: one serving

¾ cup apple juice
¼ cup Edensoy Original Soy Beverage
⅛ teaspoon ground cinnamon (optional)
½ cup Quaker Old Fashioned Oats (cooks in five minutes)
2 tablespoons golden raisins or dried apple pieces (optional)
Sugar substitute (optional)

In a saucepan, over high heat, combine apple juice, soy beverage, and optional cinnamon. Bring to a boil. Add the oats and bring mixture back to a boil. Cook for 5 minutes, stirring constantly and gradually reducing the heat. Stir in optional raisins or apple pieces and sweeten with sugar substitute if needed.

For thicker oatmeal, use a slightly heaping half cup of oats.

In a hurry? Instant oatmeal can be improved as well, by mixing in 1 part soy beverage to one part apple juice, instead of water. Microwave as per directions on label. Garnish as above.

Nutrition Totals Per Serving

Kilocalorie breakdown: 10.7% protein, 74.7% carbohydrate, 14.6% fat
Calories: 200
Protein: 5.1 (g)
Carbohydrate: 35.4 (g)
Fat: 3.1 (g)
Cholesterol: 0 (mg)
Sodium: 40 (mg)

○ Bagel Nosh

Yield: four servings

2 Lender's Large Honey Wheat Bagels
½ cup Kraft Whipped Cream Cheese (plain or chive)
8 Lightlife Smart Deli Meatless Country Ham Style Slices
8 Lightlife Smart Deli Meatless Roast Turkey Style Slices
4 slices large ripe tomato
4 slices onion

Slice or pull the bagels in half and lay them open. Spread 2 tablespoons cream cheese on each bagel half (toasted if desired), followed by 2 slices "ham," 2 slices "turkey," and a slice each of onion and tomato. Serve open face.

Nutrition Totals Per Serving

Kilocalorie breakdown: 28.4% protein, 45.1% carbohydrate, 26.5% fat
Calories: 272
Protein: 19.3 (g)
Carbohydrate: 30.7 (g)
Fat: 8.0 (g)
Cholesterol: 25 (mg)
Sodium: 760 (mg)

○ Egg n' Muffin

Yield: four servings

4 triple-layer paper muffin cups (do not use foil)
olive-oil cooking spray
1 cup Egg Beaters Real Egg Substitute (prepared as below)
4 Thomas's Oat Bran English Muffins
2½ tablespoons (8 teapoons) Land O' Lakes Light Whipped Butter (optional)
4 slices Borden's Fat Free American Singles
4 slices Yves Canadian Veggie Bacon

To cook the egg patties, coat all four of the triple-layer muffin cups with olive-oil cooking spray. Place two of them on a microwave-safe plate 3 inches apart. Pour ¼ cup egg substitute into each cup, cover with a paper towel, wax paper, or plastic wrap, and microwave on high for 1 minute. Turn the plate one quarter turn and cook for another 45 to 60 seconds. Repeat with the two remaining cups.

Lay open the muffins and spread each half with 1 teaspoon butter (if using). Peel the egg "patties" out of the paper cups and place one on the bottom half of each muffin. Cover with 1 slice cheese and 1 slice "bacon." Close the sandwich and wrap each one in a paper towel. Microwave for 30 seconds to melt the cheese and heat the bacon.

For breakfast on the go, make these ahead of time. Cover them in plastic wrap instead of a paper towel and refrigerate till ready to use (up to 3 days). Then wrap in wax paper and reheat muffins in the microwave for 30 to 60 seconds on high. The wrapper will be hot.

VARIATION: Sausage muffins are an easy alternative: Simply prepare Morningstar Farms Breakfast Patties and use one per sandwich instead of the Canadian Veggie Bacon.

Nutritional Totals Per Serving

Kilocalorie breakdown: 31.7% protein, 56.7% carbohydrate, 11.6% fat
Calories: 240
Protein: 20.3 (g)
Carbohydrate: 36.3 (g)

Fat: 3.3 (g)
Cholesterol: 7 (mg)
Sodium: 838 (mg)

SALADS AND DRESSINGS

○ Big Max Special Sauce

Yield: six servings, each two tablespoons

½ cup Nasoya Nayonaise

2 tablespoons Heinz Ketchup

2 tablespoons Heinz Sweet Pickle Relish

Combine all the ingredients in a small dish and mix till thoroughly blended. Chill and serve.

Nutrition Totals Per Serving

Kilocalorie breakdown: 0.8% protein, 22.1% carbohydrate, 77.1% fat
Calories: 57 (g)
Protein: 0.1 (g)
Carbohydrate: 2.6 (g)
Fat: 4.0 (g)
Cholesterol: 0 (mg)
Sodium: 229 (mg)

○ Chef's Salad

Yield: four servings

2 triple-layer paper muffin cups (do not use foil)

Olive-oil cooking spray

½ cup Eggbeaters Real Egg Substitute (prepared as below)

3 cups torn romaine leaves

3 cups torn iceberg lettuce

4 Lightlife Meatless Smart Deli Country Ham Style Slices, cut into thin strips

4 Lightlife Meatless Smart Deli Roast Turkey Style Slices, cut into thin strips
½ cup Healthy Choice Low Fat Shredded Cheddar Cheese
2 slices Sargento Reduced Fat Deli Style Swiss Cheese (cut into small squares, approximately ½ cup)
2 Morningstar Farms Breakfast Strips (cooked according to package instructions and crumbled into small pieces)
1 cup shredded carrot
1 small green pepper, cut into thin strips
3 whole scallions, sliced
¾ cup Kraft Light Done Right Salad Dressing (Catalina, Red Wine Vinaigrette, or Ranch)
8 tomato wedges
1 cup fat-free croutons

To make the hard-cooked egg, coat both triple-layer baking cups with olive oil cooking spray and place on a microwave-safe plate. Pour ¼ cup liquid egg into each cup, cover with a paper towel, wax paper, or plastic wrap, and microwave on high for 60 seconds. Turn plate one quarter turn and microwave for another 30 to 45 seconds. When cool enough to handle, remove the egg patties from the paper and dice them into small squares.

In a large bowl, toss together the lettuce leaves. Add all the other ingredients except the dressing, tomatoes, and croutons, and gently mix to combine. Pour on the dressing and toss to coat. Divide into 4 bowls or plates. Garnish with 2 tomato wedges per salad, ¼ cup croutons, and freshly ground black pepper if desired.

VARIATION: To offer a choice of dressings, divide undressed salad into four bowls and pass several different Kraft Light Done Right Flavors. Use 3 tablespoons per serving.

Nutritional Totals Per Serving (With Catalina Dressing)

Kilocalorie breakdown: 28.7% protein, 36.2% carbohydrate, 35.1% fat
Calories: 306
Protein: 21.7 (g)
Carbohydrate: 27.4 (g)
Fat: 11.8 (g)
Cholesterol: 8 (mg)
Sodium: 1,142 (mg)

○ Creamy Parmesan Dressing and Dip

Yield: six servings, each three tablespoons

¾ cup Nasoya Nayonaise
¼ cup reduced fat sour cream
2 teaspoons white wine vinegar
¼ teaspoon dried basil, crushed with a mortar and pestle
⅛ teaspoon garlic powder
3 tablespoons Soyco Lite and Less Veggy Parmesan Cheese Alternative
2 tablespoons Edensoy Original Soy Beverage

In a small bowl, stir together all the ingredients. Chill. Serve over mixed greens.

> *VARIATION: If making a dip, omit the soy beverage, and serve with fresh-cut vegetables or as a dipping choice for Chick "En" Nuggets (page 189).*

Nutrition Totals Per Serving

Kilocalorie breakdown: 6.3% carbohydrate, 7.7% protein, 86.0% fat
Calories: 90
Protein: 1.4 (g)
Carbohydrate: 1.2 (g)
Fat: 7.1 (g)
Cholesterol: 3 (mg)
Sodium: 298 (mg)

○ Haas Hummus

Yield: six servings, serving size approx. ⅓ cup

1 16-ounce package Fantastic Foods Original Hummus
2 teaspoons Bertolli Extra Light Olive Oil
1½ cups water
2 tablespoons Minute Maid Lemon Juice (or fresh squeezed)

Place hummus mix in a bowl. Add the water, lemon juice, and 2 teaspoons olive oil (not 2 tablespoons as called for in package directions). Stir until well blended with a wire whisk or a hand blender. Let sit for several minutes before serving. Store in the refrigerator. Serve with Hol Grain Rice Crackers or whole-wheat pita bread.

Nutrition Totals Per Serving

Kilocalorie breakdown: 13.0% protein, 48.4% carbohydrate; 38.6% fat
Calories: 135
Protein: 4.5 (g)
Carbohydrate: 16.9 (g)
Fat: 6.0 (g)
Cholesterol: 0 (mg)
Sodium: 420 (mg)

○ Mediterranean Pasta Salad

Yield: six servings

Salad:
2 heaping cups uncooked fusilli or rotini pasta
4 slices (4 ounces) Sargento Reduced Fat Deli Style Swiss Cheese, cut into small squares
1 package (5.5 ounces) Yves Veggie Pepperoni, cut into ½-inch strips
1 15-ounce can chickpeas (approximately 1½ cups)
1½ cups thinly sliced zucchini
1 cup cubed red pepper
1 small onion, cut into thin rings
¼ cup Soyco Lite & Less Veggy Parmesan Cheese Alternative
2 medium tomatoes, cut into wedges (optional)
Dressing:
3 tablespoons Bertolli Extra Light Olive Oil
⅓ cup Nasoya Nayonaise
¼ cup red wine vinegar
2 cloves garlic, minced
2 teaspoons dried basil, crushed with a mortar and pestle
1 teaspoon dried oregano, crushed
½ teaspoon freshly ground black pepper

Cook pasta according to package directions. Drain and rinse with cold water. Set aside.

To make the salad, in a large bowl combine the pasta, Swiss cheese, Veggie Pepperoni, chickpeas, zucchini, red pepper, onion slices, and Parmesan alternative. Toss to combine.

To make the dressing, combine in a jar the oil, Nayonaise, vinegar, garlic, basil, oregano, and pepper. Cover and shake vigorously. Pour over the salad ingredients. Toss to coat. Cover and chill overnight for best flavor. Add tomatoes right before serving, as they will lose texture if refrigerated.

Nutrition Totals Per Serving

Kilocalorie breakdown: 23.8% protein, 42.9% carbohydrate, 33.3% fat
Calories: 369
Protein: 21.1 (g)
Carbohydrate: 37.9 (g)
Fat: 13.1 (g)
Cholesterol: 10 (mg)
Sodium: 43.1 (mg)

○ Power-Packed Tuna Salad

Yield: four servings, ½ cup each

1 12-ounce can solid white albacore tuna, packed in spring water
½ cup Nasoya Nayonaise
½ cup diced celery

Drain and flake the tuna. Add the Nayonaise and celery, and stir to combine. Chill. Use for sandwiches or serve on a bed of lettuce as a salad with rice crackers on the side.

Nutrition Totals Per Serving

Kilocalorie breakdown: 23.8% protein, 42.9% carbohydrate, 33.3% fat
Calories: 369
Protein: 21.1 (g)
Carbohydrate: 37.9 (g)
Fat: 13.1 (g)
Cholesterol: 10 (mg)
Sodium: 43.1 (mg)

○ Spicy Mayo

Yield: eight servings, each two tablespoons

　　1 cup Nasoya Nayonaise
　　2 teaspoons Creole seasoning

In a small bowl, combine the two ingredients and stir till blended. Cover and chill.

This is used on the Chik Fillet Sandwich (page 190). Try it on sandwiches made with Yves or Lightlife Deli Slices as well.

Nutrition Totals Per Serving

　　Kilocalorie breakdown: 0% protein, 12.9% carbohydrate, 87.1% fat
　　Calories: 70
　　Protein: 0 (g)
　　Carbohydrate: 0 (g)
　　Fat: 6 (g)
　　Cholesterol: 0 (mg)
　　Sodium: 210 (mg)

SANDWICHES AND SNACKS

○ Big Max Burgers

Yield: four burgers

　　4 Morningstar Farms Harvest Burgers (Original Flavor)
　　4 hamburger buns (whole-grain if available)
　　8 tablespoons *Big Max Special Sauce* (page 181)
　　4 teaspoons dried onion flakes
　　4 Borden's Fat-Free American Singles
　　Shredded lettuce

Cook the "hamburger" patties according to package directions and set them aside. Lay the buns open and spread 1 tablespoon Big Max Special Sauce onto each bun half. Sprinkle ½ teaspoon onion flakes on each half. Lay 1 slice cheese on the bottom half of each bun. Place the "hamburger" patties on the cheese, cover them with lettuce, and close the sandwiches. To melt the cheese, wrap each "burger" in a paper towel, put them all in the microwave, and microwave on high for 20 to 30 seconds.

Serve with Fabulous French Fries (page 193), if desired.

Nutrition Totals

Kilocalorie breakdown: 35.6% protein, 38.4% carbohydrate, 25.9% fat
Calories: 315
Protein: 27.8 (g)
Carbohydrate: 30.0 (g)
Fat: 9 (g)
Cholesterol: 0 (mg)
Sodium: 1,071 (mg)

○ Classic Baked Potatoes

Yield: four servings

4 large baking potatoes
4 tablespoons Land O'Lakes Light Whipped Butter
4 tablespoons reduced-fat sour cream
4 teaspoons horseradish (optional)
4 Morningstar Farms Breakfast Strips (cooked according to package instructions and crumbled or diced)
1 cup Healthy Choice Low Fat Shredded Cheddar Cheese
4 teaspoons chopped chives (fresh or freeze-dried)
Salt and freshly ground black pepper to taste

Bake the potatoes in a 400° F. oven for 1 hour or until tender. Slice each one open lengthwise and mash pulp with a fork. Top each potato as follows:

For each potato:
1 tablespoon butter
1 teaspoon horseradish (if using)
1 tablespoon sour cream
Salt and freshly ground black pepper
(continued)

1 diced "bacon" strip

¼ cup Cheddar

1 teaspoon chopped chives

Nutrition Totals Per Serving

Kilocalorie breakdown: 28.4% protein, 29.3% carbohydrate, 42.3% fat

Calories: 280

Protein: 13.1 (g)

Carbohydrate: 13.5 (g)

Fat: 8.7 (g)

Cholesterol: 15 (mg)

Sodium: 416 (mg)

O Chicago-Style "Red Hot" Dogs

Yield: four servings

4 Morningstar Farms Veggie Dogs (preferred) or Yves Tofu Wieners

4 hot dog buns (with poppy seeds if available)

¼ cup yellow mustard

4 dill pickle slices (cut lengthwise for sandwiches)

¼ cup chopped tomato

¼ cup chopped onion

Onion salt (optional)

4 pepperoncini (optional)

Cook the veggie dogs according to package directions, preferably by simmering them in hot water. Steam the buns and lay them open face. Fill each in the following order:

1 tablespoon mustard

1 pickle slice

1 Veggie Dog

Dash onion salt (if using)

1 tablespoon chopped tomato

1 tablespoon chopped onion

1 pepperoncini (if using)

Serve with Cajun French Fries (page 193), if desired.

Nutritional Totals Per Serving

Kilocalorie breakdown: 30.1% protein, 55.1% carbohydrate, 14.7% fat
Calories: 218
Protein: 16.9 (g)
Carbohydrate: 30.8 (g)
Fat: 3.7 (g)
Cholesterol: 0 (mg)
Sodium: 1,071 (mg)

○ Chick "En" Nuggets

Yield: four servings, each four nuggets

1 package Morningstar Farms Chik Nuggets (cooked according to package directions)
½ cup Heinz Ketchup
½ cup French's Honey Mustard

Serve each plate of nuggets accompanied by 2 tablespoons ketchup and 2 tablespoons honey mustard in small dishes for dipping.

Variations: For extra-rich, creamy dipping sauces, stir in 2 tablespoons Nasoya Nayonaise to each half cup of ketchup and honey mustard. Other good dipping sauces include Spicy Mayo (page 186) and Creamy Parmesan Dressing Dip (page 183), as well as barbeque sauce and honey.

Nutrition Totals

Kilocalorie breakdown: 33.3% protein, 43.6% carbohydrate, 23.1% fat
Calories: 160
Protein: 13.0 (g)
Carbohydrate: 17.0 (g)
Fat: 4.0 (g)
Sodium: 670 (mg)
Cholesterol: 0 (mg)

○ Chik Fillet Sandwich

Yield: four servings

½ recipe (8 tablespoons) Spicy Mayo (page 186)
4 Morningstar Farms Chik Patties
4 hamburger buns (whole-grain if available)
8 leaves lettuce

Prepare the Spicy Mayo, cover, and refrigerate.

Cook the "chicken" patties according to package directions, preferably by the conventional oven method.

Lay the buns open and spread 1 tablespoon Spicy Mayo on each bun half. Place two lettuce leaves on each bun bottom, followed by a "chicken" patty and the top half of the bun.

The buns can be toasted before adding the mayonnaise spread; set them open-faced on a separate cookie sheet during the last few minutes of conventional oven baking.

Nutrition Totals Per Serving
Kilocalorie breakdown: 18.2% protein, 43.0% carbohydrate, 38.8% fat
Calories: 307
Protein: 13.7 (g)
Carbohydrate: 32.4 (g)
Fat: 13.0 (g)
Cholesterol: 0 (mg)
Sodium: 931 (mg)

○ Cordon Bleu Chik Fillet Sandwich

Yield: four sandwiches

4 Morningstar Farms Chik Patties
8 Lightlife Smart Deli Meatless Country Ham Style Slices
4 slices Sargento Light Deli Style Swiss Reduced Fat Cheese (approx. 4″ x 4″ square piece)
4 kaiser rolls (whole-grain if available)

8 tablespoons French's Honey Mustard

1 cup shredded lettuce

Cook the "chicken" patties according to package directions, preferably by the conventional oven method.

During the last few minutes of baking, place 2 slices "ham" and 1 slice cheese on each patty. (If using a microwave, add the cheese and "ham" during the last 20 seconds or so of heating.)

Lay the rolls open and spread each half with 1 tablespoon honey mustard. Lift the patties onto the bottom half of each roll. Cover with ¼ cup lettuce and the top of the roll.

The rolls can be toasted (before adding the honey mustard) by setting them open-faced on a separate cookie sheet during the last few minutes of conventional oven baking.

Nutrition Totals Per serving

Kilocalorie breakdown: 25.0% protein, 49.3% carbohydrate, 25.7% fat
Calories: 283
Protein: 16.4 (g)
Carbohydrate: 32.3 (g)
Fat: 7.5 (g)
Cholesterol: 2 (mg)
Sodium: 1,016 (mg)

○ Double Stuffed Tacos

Yield: eight tacos, two per serving

2 cups Yves Veggie Ground Round (Original Flavor) or 2 cups Browned Ground Boca Burger Recipe Basics

1 packet taco seasoning (reduced sodium if available)

8 crisp corn taco shells

8 taco-size (6-inch) low-fat flour tortillas

1 cup Taco Bell Home Originals Fat Free Refried Beans

½ cup Healthy Choice Low Fat Shredded Cheddar Cheese

½ cup taco sauce

1 cup diced tomato
1 cup shredded lettuce
½ cup low-fat sour cream

In a large skillet over medium heat, combine the veggie ground round with the taco seasoning and ¾ cup water until hot and well blended. Heat the corn taco shells in a 300 degree oven on a cookie sheet for 3 to 5 minutes. While the corn shells are baking, spread each flour tortilla with 2 tablespoons of refried beans and top with one tablespoon shredded cheddar. Remove the corn shells from the oven and place each one open side up on top of a bean-and-cheese-covered flour tortilla. Fold up the sides of the tortilla so that they cover the outside of the corn shell. Fill each crisp corn taco shell with ¼ cup "beef" mixture and 1 tablespoon taco sauce. Garnish with 2 tablespoons each tomato and lettuce and top with 1 tablespoon sour cream.

For softer flour tortillas, heat them in the microwave ahead of time. Sprinkle each tortilla with water and place between two paper towels. Stack up all the flour tortillas. Heat on high for 20 to 30 seconds. Tortillas will be very hot.

Nutritional Totals Per Serving

Kilocalorie breakdown: 20.8% protein, 62.9% carbohydrate, 16.3% fat
Calories: 424
Protein: 20.2 (g)
Carbohydrate: 61.2 (g)
Fat: 7.1 (g)
Cholesterol: 11 (mg)
Sodium: 1,449 (mg)

○ Eat to Win Chili Dogs

Yield: four sandwiches

2 cups No Alarm Chili (page 201)
4 Yves Tofu Wieners (preferred) or Lightlife Smart Dogs or Morningstar Farms Veggie
    Dogs
4 hot dog buns (whole-grain if available)
Chopped onion and/or shredded low-fat cheddar cheese

Prepare the chili. Heat the "hot dogs" according to package instructions. Toast the buns if desired and spread ¼ cup chili on each bun. Top with a hot dog and another ¼ cup chili. Garnish with chopped onion and/or shredded low-fat cheddar cheese.

Nutritional Totals Per Serving

Kilocalorie breakdown: 45.7% protein, 40.8% carbohydrate, 13.5% fat
Calories: 254
Protein: 22.1 (g)
Carbohydrate: 26.7 (g)
Fat: 4.0 (g)
Cholesterol: 0 (mg)
Sodium: 849 (mg)

○ Fabulous French Fries

Yield: six servings

1 20-ounce package Simply Potatoes New Potato Wedges or 4 cups wedge-cut new
    potatoes
2 teaspoons Bertolli Extra Light Olive Oil
1 tablespoon Eggbeaters Real Egg Substitute
2 tablespoons cornstarch
½ teaspoon salt
Olive-oil cooking spray

Preheat oven to 425° F. Place the potato wedges in a medium-size bowl. Add the oil and toss to coat, add the egg and toss again. Sprinkle on the cornstarch and salt and gently toss until the white powder is absorbed.

Line a large baking sheet with foil, and coat it with olive-oil cooking spray. Place the wedges skin side down on the sheet and bake for 15 to 20 minutes or until slightly golden and crisp tender. Serve with Heinz ketchup.

VARIATION: *For Cajun French Fries, add 1 tablespoon Creole seasoning after adding the salt and toss a final time before baking.*

Nutrition Totals Per Serving

    Kilocalorie breakdown: 9.6% protein, 74.5% carbohydrate, 15.8% fat
    Calories: 87
    Protein: 2.0 (g)
    Carbohydrate: 15.7 (g)
    Fat: 1.5 (g)
    Cholesterol: 0 (mg)
    Sodium: 259 (mg)

○ Fried "Bologna" Sandwiches

Yield: four servings

    4 teaspoons Bertolli's Extra Light Olive Oil
    16 slices Yves Veggie Deli Slices (approximately 1½ packages)
    4 6-inch pita bread rounds
    Yellow mustard
    Baby carrot sticks (optional)

Heat 1 teaspoon of the oil in a skillet and add 4 Deli Slices. Cook them till they start to curl and brown slightly, flipping them once or twice. Set the slices aside as they are finished. Repeat 3 more times, heating a teaspoon of oil each time before you add the slices.

Sprinkle the pitas with water and place each between two paper towels. Microwave 1 at a time for 20 to 30 seconds on high. When cool enough to handle, spread with mustard, lay 4 slices of "bologna" on top, and fold bread closed. Fasten with a toothpick. Serve with baby carrot sticks, if desired.

Nutrition Totals Per Serving

    Kilocalorie breakdown: 35.4% protein, 43% carbohydrate, 21.6% fat
    Calories: 214
    Protein: 18.9 (g)
    Carbohydrate: 22.9 (g)
    Fat: 5.1 (g)
    Cholesterol: 0 (mg)
    Sodium: 741 (mg)

○ Parmesan Chik Fillet Sandwich

Yield: four servings

4 Morningstar Farms Chik Patties
1 cup Sargento Shredded Light Italian Cheese Blend
4 teaspoons Soyco Lite and Less Veggy Parmesan Cheese Alternative
Pinch dried oregano
4 kaiser rolls (multi-grain if available)
8 tablespoons Ragu Pizza Sauce

Cook the "chicken" patties according to package directions, preferably by the conventional oven method.

During the last 5 minutes of baking, top each patty with ¼ cup shredded cheese, 1 teaspoon Parmesan substitute, and a pinch of oregano. (It may be necessary to remove the patties from the oven to do this safely.) If using a microwave, add the toppings during the last 20 seconds or so of heating.

Lay the rolls open and spread each half with 1 tablespoon pizza sauce. Put the patties on the bottom half of each roll. Cover with the tops and serve.

Nutrition Totals Per Serving

Kilocalorie breakdown: 28.0% protein, 41.4% carbohydrate, 30.6% fat
Calories: 328
Protein: 23.3 (g)
Carbohydrate: 34.5 (g)
Fat: 11.3 (g)
Cholesterol: 10 (mg)
Sodium: 940 (mg)

○ Pretty Peppy Party Pizzas

Yield: eight pizzas, serving four

4 Thomas's Oat Bran English Muffins
8 tablespoons Ragu Pizza Sauce
2 cups Sargento Light Shredded Italian Cheese Blend
32 slices Yves Veggie Pizza Pepperoni
4 teaspoons Soyco Light and Less Veggy Parmesan Cheese Alternative
Pinches dried oregano

Split the muffins in half and place the halves open face up. Add the toppings on each half as follows:

For each muffin half:

1 tablespoon pizza sauce

8 slices pepperoni

¼ cup shredded cheese

½ teaspoon Parmesan alternative

Pinch of oregano

Microwave all 4 muffin pizzas at a time on a microwave-safe plate on high for 60 to 90 seconds, or until the cheese melts completely.

Variation: The pizzas can also be cooked in a conventional oven. Heat them on a baking sheet for 5 minutes at 350° F and finish under the broiler.

Nutrition Totals

Kilocalorie breakdown: 36.9% protein, 38.4% carbohydrate, 24.8% fat

Calories: 327

Protein: 21.1 (g)

Carbohydrate: 28.5 (g)

Fat: 10.5 (g)

Cholesterol: 41 (mg)

Sodium: 774 (mg)

○ Totally Tuna Melts

Yield: four servings, each two muffin halves

1 recipe Power-Packed Tuna Salad (page 185)

4 Thomas's Oat Bran English Muffins

2 cups Healthy Choice Low Fat Shredded Cheddar Cheese

Prepare the tuna salad.

Split the muffins and place a ¼-cup mound of tuna on each half. Cover with ¼ cup cheese. Press cheese into tuna so that it stays in place. Microwave 2 halves at a time on a microwave-safe plate on high for one minute or until cheese melts completely.

Variation: These melts can also be made in a conventional oven. Heat the sand-wiches on a baking sheet for 5 minutes at 350° F and finish under the broiler.

Nutritional Totals Per Serving

Kilocalorie breakdown: 43.4% protein, 28.9% carbohydrate, 27.8% fat
Calories: 418
Protein: 42.8 (g)
Carbohydrate: 28.6 (g)
Fat: 12.2 (g)
Cholesterol: 35 (g)
Sodium: 1,206 (g)

SKILLET AND ONE-PAN MEALS

○ Eat to Win Beany Weenies

Yield: four servings

4 Yves Tofu Wieners (preferred) or Lightlife Smart Dogs or Morningstar Farms Veggie
　Dogs
2 Morningstar Farms Breakfast Strips, thawed at room temperature
2 tablespoons yellow mustard
2 tablespoons honey
2 tablespoons Heinz Ketchup
Olive-oil cooking spray
¼ cup chopped onion (optional)
2 16-ounce cans Heinz Vegetarian Baked Beans

Slice the "hot dogs" into small circles and dice the Breakfast Strips. Set them aside. Combine the mustard, honey, and ketchup in a small bowl and mix till uniform in color.

Coat a large skillet with olive-oil cooking spray and set over medium-high heat. Add the onion (if using) and sauté in 2 teaspoons water until the edges start to turn golden in color. Add the beans and the condiment mixture and stir to combine. Add the "hot dog" and breakfast strip pieces and stir often while heating the mixture.

Nutrition Totals Per Serving

Kilocalorie breakdown: 23.7% protein, 70.4% carbohydrate, 6.0% fat
Calories: 348
Protein: 20.1 (g)
Carbohydrate: 59.6 (g)
Fat: 2.3 (g)
Cholesterol: 0 (mg)
Sodium: 183 (mg)

○ Kidwiches (Sloppy Joes)

Yield: six servings

1 15½-ounce can Hunt's Manwich Sauce (regular or barbecue flavor)
1 package (2 cups) Yves Veggie Ground Round (original flavor) or 2 cups Browned Ground
    Boca Burger Recipe Basics
6 hamburger buns
Baby carrot sticks (optional)

Pour the Manwich Sauce into a large skillet set over medium heat and crumble the ground round into it. Stir to combine. When thoroughly heated, spoon a generous portion onto the bottom half of each bun. Cover with the tops and serve alongside baby carrot sticks, if desired.

Nutrition Totals Per Serving

Kilocalorie breakdown: 36.2% protein, 58.9% carbohydrate, 4.9% fat
Calories: 181
Protein: 1,616 (g)
Carbohydrate: 27.0 (g)
Fat: 1.0 (g)
Cholesterol: 0 (mg)
Sodium: 823 (mg)

○ Krafty Carbonara (Hay and Straw)

Yield: three servings

1 7¼-ounce box Kraft's Macaroni and Cheese Dinner (Cheesy Alfredo Flavor)
2 tablespoons Land O' Lakes Light Whipped Butter

⅓ cup Edensoy Original Soy Beverage
½ cup Green Giant Select Baby Sweet Peas
3 slices Yves Canadian Veggie Bacon (thinly sliced strips, Julienne-style)
Cracked black pepper

Prepare the Macaroni and Cheese Dinner according to package directions, substituting the 2 tablespoons light butter for the margarine and the soy beverage for the milk. (Add the peas during the last 2 minutes of cooking the pasta. Stir in the sliced "bacon" along with the cheese powder, butter, and soy beverage.) Keep stirring until the sauce thickens. Season with cracked black pepper.

Nutrition Totals Per Serving

Kilocalorie breakdown: 21.8% protein, 64.0% carbohydrate, 14.2% fat
Calories: 348
Protein: 18.9 (g)
Carbohydrate: 55.6 (g)
Fat: 5.5 (g)
Cholesterol: 17 (mg)
Sodium: 844 (mg)

◯ Krafty Macaroni and Cheese

Yield: three servings

1 7¼-ounce box Kraft Macaroni and Cheese Dinner
3 tablespoons Land O'Lakes Light Whipped Butter
¼ cup Edensoy Original Soy Beverage
1 cup steamed broccoli florets (optional)

Prepare the Macaroni and Cheese Dinner according to package directions, substituting the 3 tablespoons light butter for the margarine and the soy beverage for the milk.

For extra goodness, add 1 cup steamed broccoli florets to the mixture.

Variation on Kraft's Instant Dinner: Soy milk can improve the nutrition of Kraft Easy Mac instant macaroni and cheese as well. Use Westsoy 1% lite instead of water when microwaving the pasta. Reduce heating time to 2½ minutes (keep an eye

*on the bowl to make sure it doesn't boil over). Stir in 1 teaspoon Land O'Lakes
Light Whipped Butter along with the cheese powder.*

Nutrition Totals Per Serving

Kilocalorie breakdown: 14.2% protein, 68.5% carbohydrate, 17.3% fat
Calories: 306
Protein: 11.8 (g)
Carbohydrate: 57.0 (g)
Fat: 6.4 (g)
Cholesterol: 20 (mg)
Sodium: 614 (mg)

○ New Brunswick Stew

Yield: four servings

2 15-ounce cans Health Valley Mild Vegetarian Chili With Lentils
6 Yves Veggie Breakfast Links, sliced
1 cup Green Giant Extra Sweet Corn (frozen or canned)
¼ cup ketchup

Combine the ingredients together in a saucepan and cook over medium heat
until hot.

Nutritional Totals Per Serving

Kilocalorie breakdown: 36.2% protein, 63.3% carbohydrate, 0.5% fat
Calories: 248
Protein: 23.7 (g)
Carbohydrate: 41.5 (g)
Fat: 0.2 (g)
Cholesterol: 18 (mg)
Sodium: 616 (mg)

○ No Alarm Chili

Yield: four servings

Olive-oil cooking spray
⅓ cup diced onion (optional)
14½-ounce can Del Monte Fresh Cut Diced Tomatoes (no salt added)
1 package Yves Veggie Ground Round (Original Flavor), or 2 cups Browned Ground Boca
    Burger Recipe Basics
15½-ounce can Bush's Chili Magic (any flavor)

Coat a saucepan with olive-oil cooking spray and sauté the onion (if using) in 2 teaspoons water until tender. Add the undrained tomatoes, veggie ground round, and chili mix to the pan. Mix together and cook over medium heat 20 to 30 minutes, stirring occasionally. The chili will get thicker and more flavorful the longer it's cooked.

Serve with your choice of low-fat or fat-free versions of classic chili toppings like sour cream and shredded cheddar cheese, plus oyster crackers and chopped onion.

Nutritional Totals Per Serving

Kilocalorie breakdown: 55.6% protein, 35.6% carbohydrate, 8.8% fat
Calories: 234
Protein: 21.0 (g)
Carbohydrate: 13.5 (g)
Fat: 1.5 (g)
Cholesterol: 0 (mg)
Sodium: 1,416 (mg)

ENTRÉES

○ Italian Stuffed Peppers

Yield: four servings

2 cups cooked brown rice (Success Rice Boil in Bags can be prepared in 10 minutes)
4 large green bell peppers

1 package Yves Veggie Ground Round or 2 cups Browned Ground Boca Burger Recipe
    Basics
1 26-ounce jar Classico Pasta Sauce (Roasted Peppers and Onions)
½ cup Egg Beaters Real Egg Substitute
1 teaspoon garlic powder
1 tablespoon dried onion flakes
½ teaspoon salt
2 tablespoons Soyco Lite and Less Veggy Parmesan Cheese Alternative

Preheat the oven to 350° F. Prepare the rice.

Rinse the peppers, remove the stems, and cut them in half lengthwise. Remove the ribs and seeds. Place the peppers open face up, covered by paper towels, on a large microwave-safe plate. Heat them on 50% power for 10 minutes. You could also boil them in a large pot on the stove for 3 minutes.

In a large bowl, combine the veggie ground round, rice, 1/2 cup of the pasta sauce, the egg substitute, garlic powder, onion flakes, and salt. Mix thoroughly.

Coat a large baking pan (about 10 by 13 inches) with olive-oil cooking spray. Pour half the remaining jar of pasta sauce into the pan and spread it out to cover the bottom. Divide the stuffing mixture among the 8 pepper halves by filling them one at a time and arranging them open face up in the prepared baking pan. Drizzle the remaining sauce over the peppers and sprinkle with Parmesan cheese alternative. Bake for 25 to 30 minutes. When serving, scoop the pasta sauce over the peppers.

Nutrition Totals Per Serving

Kilocalorie breakdown: 31.8% protein, 57.2% carbohydrate, 11.0 fat
Calories: 352
Protein: 28.4 (g)
Carbohydrate: 51.2 (g)
Fat: 4.4 (g)
Cholesterol: 0.0 (mg)
Sodium: 1,689 (mg)

○ Lemon "Chicken"

Yield: four servings

2 cups brown rice (Success Rice Boil in Bags can be prepared in 10 minutes)

24 (about 1½ packages) Morningstar Farms Chik Nuggets

1 tablespoon cornstarch

1 cup Minute Maid Fresh Lemon Juice (or freshly squeezed)

2 tablespoons canola oil

¼ cup honey

¼ cup light corn syrup

2 cups parboiled Green Giant Sugar Snap Peas (optional)

Thinly sliced lemon

Prepare the rice. Cook the nuggets according to package directions, preferably by conventional oven method.

Dissolve the cornstarch in ¼ cup of the lemon juice and stir till smooth. Add to a large saucepan along with the remaining ¾ cup lemon juice, canola oil, honey, and corn syrup. Stir over medium heat until mixture starts to thicken. Add the crisped nuggets to the pan and gently mix to coat.

Place a ½ cup mound of rice in the center of each of 4 plates and ladle 6 nuggets per serving on top. Encircle each entrée with ½ cup sugar snap peas (if using). Divide the remaining lemon sauce over the 4 portions. Garnish with thin slices of fresh lemon.

Nutrition Totals Per Serving

Kilocalorie breakdown: 15.5% protein, 63.3% carbohydrate, 21.2% fat

Calories: 564

Protein: 22.5 (g)

Carbohydrate: 91.6 (g)

Fat: 13.6 (g)

Cholesterol: 0.0 (mg)

Sodium: 1,299 (mg)

◯ Linguine with "Chicken" Parmesan

Yield: four servings

4 Morningstar Farms Chik Patties
1 cup Sargento Shredded Light Italian Cheese Blend
4 teaspoons Soyco® Lite and Less Veggy Parmesan Cheese Alternative
Pinches dried oregano
8 ounces uncooked linguine
2 cups low-fat Classico Pasta Sauce (choose a flavor with no more than 4 grams of fat per ½ cup)
Fresh basil leaves (optional)

Cook the patties according to package directions, preferably by conventional oven method.

During the last 5 minutes of baking, top each patty with ¼ cup shredded cheese, 1 teaspoon Parmesan alternative, and a pinch of oregano. (It may be necessary to remove the patties from the oven to do this safely.) If microwaving them, add the toppings during the last 20 seconds of heating.

While the patties finish baking, cook the pasta till al dente, and heat the sauce. Divide the linguine evenly between 4 plates or shallow bowls. Ladle ¼ cup sauce onto each serving of linguine, and ¼ cup sauce over each fillet. Garnish with a fresh basil leaf if desired.

Nutritional Totals Per Serving

Kilocalorie breakdown: 25.1% protein, 47.7% carbohydrate, 27.2% fat
Calories: 442
Protein: 27.1 (g)
Carbohydrate: 51.6 (g)
Fat: 13.1 (g)
Cholesterol: 10 (mg)
Sodium: 1,194 (mg)

O "Meaty" Baked Ziti

Yield: four servings

2 cups uncooked ziti
2 large egg whites
2 tablespoons Soyco Lite and Less Veggy Parmesan Cheese Alternative
1 cup fat-free ricotta cheese
⅛ teaspoon cracked black pepper
1 cup plus 2 tablespoons Sargento Shredded Light Italian Cheese Blend
1½ cups Yves Veggie Ground Round (Italian flavor) or Browned Ground Boca Burger
   Recipe Basics (flavor with a little Italian seasoning)
Olive-oil cooking spray

Preheat the oven to 350° F. Cook the ziti to the al dente stage. Drain, rinse with cool water, and set aside.

In a large bowl, beat the egg whites with a fork. Add the Parmesan alternative and the pepper. Stir. Add the ricotta and Italian cheese blend, and mix well. Add the pasta and crumbled ground round, and stir to combine.

Coat a 2-quart casserole with olive-oil cooking spray. Fill it in the following order, making sure to spread out each layer as evenly as possible:

½ cup sauce
half the pasta mixture
½ cup sauce
the rest of the pasta mixture
the rest of the sauce (¾ cup)
2 tablespoons shredded cheese blend sprinkled over the top.

Cover and bake for 25 minutes. Remove the lid and bake for 5 more minutes. Let the casserole sit 5 to 10 minutes before serving.

Nutritional Totals Per Serving

Kilocalorie breakdown: 42.1% protein, 42.5% carbohydrate, 15.4% fat
Calories: 431
Protein: 43.8 (g)
Carbohydrate: 44.2 (g)
Fat: 7.1 (g)
Cholesterol: 16 (mg)
Sodium: 996 (mg)

○ Poached Salmon

Yield: four servings

Olive-oil cooking spray
1 pound salmon steaks or fillets (4 ounces each), sprinkled lightly with garlic powder
½ cup water
½ cup dry sherry
2 teaspoons Tamari soy sauce
2 lemons, thinly sliced
4 scallions (green part only), chopped

Preheat the oven to 350° F. Coat a baking pan with olive-oil cooking spray. Arrange the salmon steaks or fillets in the pan. Combine the water, sherry, and soy sauce, and pour the mixture over the salmon. Lay lemon slices on top of each steak or fillet. Cover with lid or foil. Bake 45 to 60 minutes. Uncover for the last 10 minutes of baking and sprinkle with the scallions.

Serve with Classic Baked Potatoes, if desired (page 187), and a steamed vegetable of choice.

Nutrition Totals Per Serving

Kilocalorie breakdown: 52% protein, 17% carbohydrate, 31% fat
Calories: 217
Protein: 27.7 (g)
Carbohydrate: 8.9 (g)
Fat: 7.7 (g)
Cholesterol: 47 (mg)
Sodium: 190 (mg)

○ Spaghettini Bolognese (with "Meat" Sauce)

Yield: four servings

26-ounce jar low-fat Classico Pasta Sauce (4 grams of fat per half cup or less; Pecorino Romano and Herb is recommended)
1 cup Yves Veggie Ground Round (Italian Flavor) or Browned Ground Boca Burger Recipe Basics (flavor with a little Italian seasoning)

1 pound uncooked spaghettini

Soyco Lite and Less Veggy Parmesan Cheese Alternative

Combine the pasta sauce with the crumbled ground round in a saucepan and bring to a simmer over medium heat.

Cook the spaghetti till al dente. Drain and distribute evenly in 4 pasta bowls. Ladle on "meat" sauce (approximately ¾ cup per serving) and sprinkle with Parmesan Cheese Alternative.

Nutrition Totals Per Serving

Kilocalorie breakdown: 21.3% protein, 69.2% carbohydrate, 9.5% fat
Calories: 578
Protein: 29.9 (g)
Carbohydrate: 97.3 (g)
Fat: 6.0 (g)
Cholesterol: 0 (mg)
Sodium: 869 (mg)

DESSERTS

○ English Trifle

Yield: four servings

12 reduced-fat vanilla wafers
1 3-ounce package Jell-O Vanilla Cook & Serve Pudding and Pie Filling
2 cups Edensoy Original Soy Beverage
8 teaspoons raspberry preserves
Ready Whip Fat Free Dairy Whipped Topping (optional)

Arrange 4 dessert dishes with 3 vanilla wafers in the bottom of each one. Set aside. Cook the pudding according to package directions, substituting the soy beverage for the milk. When the pudding starts to boil, remove it from the heat and pour an even amount into each dish—about ½ cup.

Drop 2 teaspoons preserves into the center of each pudding. If the wafers rise to the top, gently push them back down with a spoon. Let the pudding cool slightly and then refrigerate, or serve warm. Garnish with Ready Whip Fat Free Dairy Whipped Topping, if desired.

Nutrition Totals Per Serving

Kilocalorie breakdown: 10.8% protein, 73.2% carbohydrate, 16.1% fat
Calories: 231
Protein: 5.8 (g)
Carbohydrate: 39.1 (g)
Fat: 3.8 (g)
Cholesterol: 0 (mg)
Sodium: 240 (mg)

◯ Fantastic Fruit Cup

Yield: four servings

1 cup strawberries, stems removed and halved

1 cup blueberries

1 cup cubed fresh pineapple

1 cup red seedless grapes

½ cup Dannon Vanilla Flavored Low Fat Yogurt

1 tablespoon Eagle Fat Free Sweetened Condensed Milk

2 tablespoons lime juice

½ cup Ready Whip Fat Free Dairy Whipped Topping

½ teaspoon finely grated lime peel (optional)

Wash and prepare the fruit.

In a small bowl combine the yogurt, condensed milk, and lime juice and stir to blend. Fold in the whipped topping and gently stir to combine.

In a medium-size bowl, mix together all the fruit. Divide the mixture between 4 dessert dishes. Distribute the yogurt sauce evenly over the fruit (about ¼ cup per serving). Garnish with lime peel, if using. Serve immediately or cover each dish with plastic wrap and refrigerate 1 to 3 hours.

Nutrition Totals Per Serving

Kilocalorie breakdown: 7.8% protein, 84.8% carbohydrate, 7.4% fat
Calories: 132
Protein: 2.6 (g)
Carbohydrate: 27.9 (g)

Fat: 1.1 (g)
Cholesterol: 2 (mg)
Sodium: 29 (mg)

❍ Nice Crispy Treats/Breakfast Cereal Bars

Yield: 12 servings, 2 treats each or 1 Breakfast Cereal Bar

1 tablespoon plus 1 teaspoon canola oil
2 tablespoons Land O' Lakes Light Whipped Butter
1 10½-ounce package miniature marshmallows
6 cups Kellogg's Just Right Cereal Fruit & Nut
Apple wedges (optional)

Coat a $13 \times 9 \times 2$-inch pan with ½ teaspoon canola oil.

Combine 1 tablespoon oil and the butter in a large saucepan and melt over low heat. Add the marshmallows and stir until completely melted. Add the cereal and mix until coated. Transfer the mixture into the pan and press evenly with a flat object that has been lightly coated with canola oil.

Let the mixture cool; then cut it into 2-inch squares. For Breakfast Cereal Bars, cut the mixture into 2×4-inch rectangles.

Store these treats in the refrigerator. Wrap them individually in wax paper, foil, or plastic wrap for easy snacks on the go or lunchbox desserts. Serve with crisp apple wedges, if desired.

Nutrition Totals Per Treat-Size Serving

Kilocalorie breakdown: 3.6% protein, 85.2% carbohydrate, 11.2% fat
Calories: 218
Protein: 2.0 (g)
Carbohydrate: 47.4 (g)
Fat: 2.8 (g)
Cholesterol: 2 (mg)
Sodium: 148 (g)

GLOSSARY

Acetylcholine: A neurotransmitter involved primarily in memory, sensory input, and muscular movement: Acetylcholine is synthesized from the amino acid choline.

Aerobic activity: Low-intensity, high-endurance activity that requires oxygen.

Alpha-linolenic acid: An essential fatty acid found in flaxseed and a number of other plant seed oils.

Alpha-lipoic acid: Alpha-lipoic acid is a powerful antioxidant that regenerates vitamin C and vitamin E and increases glutathione levels (another antioxidant). Alpha-lipoic acid is involved in metabolism and energy production. In addition, it normalizes blood glucose levels, protects DNA from damage, and reduces the bonding of glucose with proteins in cells, which slows down aging.

Amino acid: A molecule containing ammonia and organic acids that forms the building blocks of all proteins. The human body requires twenty-two specific amino acids—twelve of them can be synthesized by the body (nonessential amino acids), whereas ten must be obtained from foods (essential amino acids).

Ammonia: A toxic metabolic waste product of protein metabolism.

Anabolism: The biochemical process in which muscle or other tissue is synthesized; a process of biologic growth.

Antioxidant: A natural or synthetic chemical or a nutrient that inactivates the damaging portion (active site) of free radicals. Antioxidants also help neutralize chemicals that cause free radical formation. Phytonutrients such as lycopene, alpha- and beta-carotene, vitamins B_1, B_5, B_6, C, E, the minerals selenium and zinc, coenzyme Q_{10}, uric acid, and three enzymes in your body (superoxide dismutase, catalase, and glutathione peroxidase) are all antioxidants. By neutralizing free radicals, antioxidants prevent damage to cell membranes and such genetic material as DNA.

Arachidonic acid: This is a 22-carbon long-chain fatty acid that promotes inflammation in bodily tissues. Arachidonic acid is found in meats and dairy products and can be manufactured by the body, especially when the diet consists of high intakes of sugar and such vegetable oils as safflower oil and corn oil.

Ascorbic acid: The chemical name for vitamin C.

Atherosclerosis: The disease process by which arteries narrow. A diet high in saturated fats and cholesterol has been implicated in causing and accelerating atherosclerosis. Elevated homocysteine (an amino acid formed during protein metabolism) levels in the blood, a result of eating a high-protein diet and/or consuming insufficient vitamin B_{12} and folic acid (both are B-vitamins), can also damage arteries and lead to atherosclerosis.

ATP (adenosine triphosphate): The universal energy molecule. ATP is synthesized in the mitochondria, organelles that metabolize protein, fat, and carbohydrate into energy, which is stored in the phosphate bonds of ATP. When ATP is split by enzymes, energy is released for various cellular functions, including muscular contraction.

Beta-carotene (pro-vitamin A): A yellowish pigment found in plants, such as carrots, squash, and pumpkin. An enzyme splits one molecule of beta-carotene in half, forming two molecules of active vitamin A. Beta-carotene is just one of at least ten carotenes found in human blood. Beta-carotene is also a power antioxidant that neutralizes a damaging type of activated oxygen called singlet oxygen.

Bioflavonoids: Bioflavonoids, found in fruits and vegetables, comprise more than 20,000 compounds that help reduce muscle soreness and inflammation, and protect the body against free radical damage.

BMI (Body Mass Index): BMI is a measure of body fatness that allows people of varying heights and weights to know if they are slender, overfat, or obese. Most fashion models and thin people have a BMI between 17 and 22. Fat people have a BMI of 25, and obese individuals have a BMI of 30 or greater. You can determine your BMI using the following formula: Divide your weight in kilograms by the square of your height in meters. If you are metrically challenged, you can calculate your BMI as follows:

1. Multiply your weight in pounds by 703.
2. Multiply your height in inches by itself.
3. Divide the first number by the second.
4. Round to the nearest whole number

BMI is not an accurate measure of body fatness for body builders, the elderly, and those who are pregnant.

Calorie: A unit of measurement used to express the energy value of food, more correctly called a kilocalorie, since it represents 1,000 times the energy of the calorie used to measure chemical reactions in a test tube. One kilocalorie is the amount of heat required to raise 1 kilogram of water (2.2 pounds) 1 degree centigrade (almost 2 degrees Fahrenheit).

Carotenoid: See **Phytonutrient.**

Conversion of Amino Acids to Catecholamines

How does eating protein wake up your brain and promote peak performance? The answer lies, in part, with the conversion of two amino acids, L-phenylalanine and L-tyrosine, to the neurotransmitters dopamine, norepinephrine, and epinephrine (commonly called adrenalin). Dopamine helps regulate muscular movement, while norepinephrine revs up the brain and epinephrine prepares the body for athletic competition. These two amino acids are found in such low-fat and protein-rich foods as tuna fish, egg whites, legumes, soy foods, and soy cocktails.

Catabolism: The biochemical process in which complex molecules are broken down for energy production, recycling of their components, or excretion.

Catecholamines: A group of brain neurotransmitters (chemicals that communicate messages between nerves), including norepinephrine and dopamine. All catecholamines are synthesized from the two amino acids L-phenylalanine and L-tyrosine.

Cell membrane: The outer boundary of a cell. Also called the plasma membrane.

Cholesterol: A sterol manufactured in the liver and other cells, found only in animal protein and fats and oils (one exception: spirulina, a blue-green algae, contains cholesterol). The body uses cholesterol to synthesize hormones and cell membranes. High levels of plasma cholesterol (called LDL) are associated with an increased risk of cardiovascular disease. Oxidized cholesterol is suspected as the primary culprit in artery damage.

Choline: Associated with the B-vitamin family, choline is converted to the neurotransmitter acetylcholine in the brain. Choline can serve as a smart nutrient, boosting memory and mental focus.

Chromium: Chromium is an element required for normal carbohydrate metabolism. Chromium helps the hormone insulin clear the blood of glucose and move it into cells.

Chromium picolinate: A special form of chromium, developed by a scientist at the U.S. Department of Agriculture, that is several times more effective than chromium. Chromium picolinate improves insulin sensitivity and helps regulate carbohydrate entry into muscle cells.

Coenzyme Q_{10}: A substance responsible for the body's synthesis of adenosine triphosphate (ATP), the universal energy molecule. Research suggests that coenzyme Q_{10} acts as a fat-soluble free-radical neutralizer and helps regulate the electrical conduction system of the heart.

Collagen: A simple protein that is one of the chief components of connective tissue.

Complete protein: An outdated nutritional concept still promoted by many nutritionists and dietitians based on the belief that only animal foods contain all 9 or 10 essential amino acids in amounts that are sufficient to maintain normal growth rate and body weight.

Cortisol: A hormone secreted by the adrenal glands during periods of stress that stimulates catabolism.

Creatine monohydrate: This compound, found in animal flesh and dietary supplements, helps replenish the body's supply of ATP (adenosine triphosphate), the universal energy molecule responsible for powering all muscular contraction and body functions. Ingesting supplementary creatine causes muscles to swell with water and increases the force of muscular contractions in activities that require short bursts of energy.

Creatinine: A metabolic byproduct of creatine metabolism.

Cysteine: A sulfur-containing amino acid with antioxidant properties.

D-alpha tocopherol: Natural vitamin E. This is the preferred form to use as a dietary supplement because it contains all of the natural isomers, or chemical forms, of vitamin E required by the body to fight diseases such as cancer and atherosclerosis.

Degenerative disease: The gradual deterioration of a biological system resulting from free-radical damage and other aging biologic processes.

DMAE (Dimethylaminoethanol): A compound found in seafood and dietary supplements (such as the **Choline Cocktail** recipe in this book) that increases the body's synthesis of acetylcholine, a neurotransmitter that helps regulate thought, memory, mental focus, and muscle contraction.

DNA: Deoxyribonucleic acid, the genetic-blueprint double-helix molecular complex in the nucleus of every cell of every living organism.

Docosahexaenoic acid (DHA): An omega-3 fatty acid found primarily in seafood and some plant seeds.

Dopamine: A neurotransmitter that controls fine movement, immune function, mood, insulin regulation, short-term memory, and emotions and drives.

Double-blind: A method of designing a scientific experiment so that neither the experimental subjects nor the investigator knows what treatment, if any, a subject is getting until after the experiment is over.

Eicosapentaenoic acid (EPA): An omega-3 fatty acid found in seafood; chemical precursors of EPA are found in seeds and nuts.

Electron transport system: The metabolic process in which electrons are passed between certain molecules and cofactors, releasing energy that is used to regenerate adenosine triphosphate (ATP) molecules.

Enzymes: Proteins that are capable of inducing chemical changes in other substances without being changed or transformed themselves.

Ergogenic: Any compound that increases the body's ability to do work. Commonly used ergogenic compounds include caffeine, fats, guaraná, carbohydrates, creatine monohydrate, phosphate salts, and choline.

Estrogen: A steroid sex hormone made from cholesterol in the body that promotes secondary female characteristics.

Flavonoids: Compounds present in fruits, vegetables, nuts, and seeds—such as flavonols, flavones, catechins, flavanones, and anthocyanins. The main dietary sources of these compounds in the U. S. diet are tea, onions, fruits, and wine. The main flavonoid in onions is quercetin glucoside, and the main flavonoid in tea is quercetin rutinoside. Flavonoid intake has been inversely linked with coronary heart disease and cancer.

Free radical: A chemically reactive atom, molecule, or molecular fragment (usually containing oxygen) generated during exercise, infection, or normal metabolic processes that can damage healthy cells and accelerate the aging process. Antioxidants, such as vitamin E, vitamin C, and coenzyme Q_{10} can quench free radicals before they damage muscles and vital organs.

Genistein: An isoflavone found in soy foods and beverages that lowers serum cholesterol and inhibits enzymes that promote tumor growth.

Ginkgo biloba: An extract from leaves of the ginkgo tree with antioxidant properties.

Gland: An group of cells that secrete a chemical or hormone.

Gluconeogenesis: When the body needs additional glucose for energy, the body synthesizes it from amino acids drawn from muscle tissue breakdown. This process, which frequently occurs during extended periods of physical activity, is known as gluconeogenesis (gluco = sugar; neo = new; genesis = creation).

Glucose: A simple carbohydrate (monosaccharide), also referred to as dextrose.

Glucose polymer: A processed form of polysaccharides, usually derived from starch, found in many sports drinks.

Glycogen: The storage form of carbohydrate fuel used by animals.

Glycogen-bound water: The water that is stored in the muscles along with glycogen. About 3 grams of water are stored with every gram of glycogen.

Glycogen depletion: The draining of the body's glycogen stores through exercise or underconsumption of carbohydrates or both.

Glycogenolysis: The metabolic process in which glycogen is broken down.

Glycogen replenishment: The replenishing of the body's glycogen stores through carbohydrate and protein consumption.

Gram: A measurement of weight equal to approximately one twenty-ninth of an ounce.

Guaraná: A South American plant that contains caffeine and caffeinelike substances.

High-density lipoproteins (HDLs): Lipoprotein carrier molecules that help prevent cholesterol buildup in the arteries.

Hormone: One of the numerous substances produced by endocrine glands and other cells that travel to other sites and regulate bodily functions.

Hydrogenation: The chemical process in which unsaturated fatty acids derived from plants are saturated with hydrogen atoms to make them more solid.

Hypertension: High blood pressure.

Incomplete protein: An outdated nutritional concept, still promoted by many nutritionists and dietitians, based on the belief that only vegetable foods are deficient in one or more of the 9 or 10 essential amino acids in amounts that are sufficient to maintain normal growth rate and body weight.

Inhibitory neurotransmitter: A neurotransmitter that decreases the electrochemical activity of neurons. GABA (gamma-aminobutyric acid) and serotonin are inhibitory neurotransmitters.

Insulin resistance: A condition in which the body becomes resistant to the effects of the glucose-regulating hormone, insulin. Adult-onset diabetes and obesity are diseases characterized by insulin resistance.

Isoflavone: A phytonutrient found in legumes and vegetables that can prevent sex hormones from stimulating cellular growth that leads to cancer. Soybeans and garbanzo beans are rich sources of isoflavones.

Ketone: An incompletely burned fatty acid produced in the liver during starvation (i.e., when carbohydrate intake is low). High-protein/low-carbohydrate diets promote the synthesis of ketones in a process called ketosis.

L-carnitine: This amino acid–like compound is required by the body to burn fat for energy. L-carnitine is found in animal flesh and can be taken as a dietary supplement. Recent studies indicate that it may increase the body's synthesis of ATP (adenosine triphosphate), the universal energy molecule.

L-glutamine: Glutamine is an amino acid that traps toxic ammonia molecules (ordinary byproducts of protein metabolism) and helps shuttle them to the kidneys, where they are excreted in urine.

Linoleic acid: An essential fatty acid found in vegetable oils and cereals and grains.

Lipolysis: The metabolic process in which triglycerides are broken down into their constituent fatty acids and glycerol. Glycerol can then be used to resynthesize glucose, and fatty acids can be burned in the body for energy.

Lipoprotein: A protein-lipid complex made in the liver that transports fat-soluble compounds (e.g., vitamins, drugs, cholesterol, and fats) in the blood.

L-methionine: A sulfur-containing amino acid with strong antioxidant properties.

L-phenylalanine: An amino acid used to synthesize the catecholamine neurotransmitters.

L-taurine: A nonessential amino acid that possesses antioxidant properties and helps stabilize the conduction of electrical impulses in the heart, nervous system, and brain.

L-tyrosine: An amino acid that serves as a precursor for the catecholamine neurotransmitters.

Lycopene: A red-pigmented phytonutrient from the carotenoid family, related to beta-carotene. Lycopene is found in such foods as watermelon, papaya, and tomatoes and is thought to reduce the risk of certain types of cancer in laboratory animals and humans.

Macronutrient: A nutrient, such as a carbohydrate, fat, or protein, required by the body in gram quantities.

Metabolic pathway: A sequence of metabolic reactions leading to byproducts and final products.

Metabolic rate: The rate at which an individual burns calories; the body's total daily caloric expenditure.

Methionine: A sulfur-containing amino acid with strong antioxidant properties.

Methylation: The combining of methyl groups (CH3-) derived from choline, S-adenosylmethionine, vitamin B_{12}, betaine, trimethylglycine (TMG), and folic acid to synthesize amino acids and control DNA activity.

Microgram (mcg): One one-millionth of a gram. A number of essential minerals, such as chromium and selenium, are consumed in microgram quantities. Most vitamins are consumed in milligram quantities (1,000 times larger).

Microtrauma: Small tears in the muscle cells due to exercise stress.

Milligram: A measurement of weight equal to 1/1,000th of a gram.

Mitochondria: The "power plants" inside cells where oxygen and nutrients are metabolized to water, carbon dioxide, and ATP.

Monosaccharide: A simple carbohydrate composed of one sugar molecule, such as glucose.

Monounsaturated fatty acid: A fatty acid that has one double bond (e.g., olive oil).

Muscle mass: Muscle tissue.

Muscle tissue: Tissue that has the ability to contract voluntarily or involuntarily: skeletal muscle, cardiac muscle, and smooth muscle.

Neuron: A nerve cell.

Neurotransmitter: A chemical substance that transmits nerve impulses between the brain and nerves, muscles, and other organs.

Nootropic: A class of nutrients or drugs that enhances mental functioning (from the Greek: *noos* = mind; *tropein* = toward).

Norepinephrine: An excitatory neurotransmitter involved in alertness, concentration, aggression, and motivation. Norepinephrine is made in the brain from the amino acids L-phenylalanine and L-tyrosine.

Orthostatic hypotension: If you've ever stood up quickly after sitting for a long time and felt dizzy, you were probably experiencing a phenomenon known as orthostatic hypotension. High-protein fad diets can also cause dizziness and fainting due to this condition. It is usually temporary and abates when you return to a moderate protein diet.

Oxidation: A chemical reaction in which an atom or molecule loses electrons or hydrogen atoms.

Phenolic: See **Phytonutrient.**

Phytochemical: A term used interchangeably with **phytonutrient.**

Phytonutrient: One of tens of thousands of compounds found in vegetables, fruits, herbs, and plants that promote good health and reduce the risk of such diseases as cancer, atherosclerosis, and type II diabetes. Phytonutrients are responsible for imparting characteristic colors, flavors, and aromas to fruits, vegetables, and herbs. Polyphenols, phenolics, carotenoids, and bioflavonoids are all examples of phytonutrients.

Placebo: An inert compound usually given to a portion of a drug study's subjects in order to distinguish the psychological effects of the experiment from the physiological effects of the drug being tested.

Polyphenol: See **Phytonutrient.**

Potassium: A mineral responsible for transmitting electrical impulses. Potassium is highly active in muscles, the brain, and neurons.

Precursor: An intermediate substance in the body's production of another substance.

Prostaglandin: A hormonelike compound, derived from linoleic acid, that regulates metabolism, inflammation, and immunity.

Quercetin: This phytonutrient possesses anti-inflammatory, antiviral, and antitumor properties. Quercetin inhibits the release of histamine and other inflammatory mediators (such as hyaluronidase and neutrophil lysosomal enzyme) from mast cells, basophils, neutrophils, and macrophages during infection and inflammation due to injury. Quercetin also inhibits many of the inflammatory products of the steps in fatty acid metabolism, especially phospholipase A2 and lipoxygenase enzyme production. Fewer inflammatory products result in reduced formation of leukotrienes (1,000 times more inflammatory than histamine), which are linked to asthma, psoriasis, gout, ulcerative colitis, and cancer.

Receptors: Sites on the outside of cells where particular molecules such as hormones can attach. This attachment to the receptor site causes corresponding changes within the cell.

Saturated fatty acid: A fatty acid that has no sites of unsaturation or double bonds. Saturated fatty acids tend to be solid at room temperature.

Selenium: An antioxidant trace mineral

Sesamin: A phytonutrient found in sesame seeds and sesame oil that possesses anti-inflammatory properties.

SOD (superoxide dismutase): A enzyme that contains copper, zinc, manganese, or iron that prevents oxygen-related free radicals (called superoxide radicals) from damaging vital organs. Superoxide dismutase catalyzes the reaction:

$$2\,O_2- + 2H^+ \rightarrow O_2 + H_2O_2$$

$O_2^- $ = superoxide ion

H^+ = hydrogen ion

H_2O_2 = hydrogen peroxide

Sports rehydration drink: A drink designed to replace the water, glucose, and electrolytes lost during vigorous physical activity and sweating.

Synergy: The action of two or more compounds combined such that their effects are greater than the sum of their individual effects.

Testosterone: A steroid sex hormone synthesized in the body from cholesterol, responsible for secondary sex characteristics in males and females. Testosterone is the parent molecule for estrogen, the predominant female steroid sex hormone.

Toxic: Poisonous. Everything, including water and oxygen, is toxic in sufficiently high doses.

Trans-fatty acids: Fatty acid typically found in foods made with hydrogenated vegetable oils that have been chemically altered to increase stability and shelf-life. Studies have linked high intake of trans-fatty acids to elevated blood cholesterol levels and increased risk of heart disease.

Triglycerides: Another name for the fat in foods and the fat synthesized by the body. Triglycerides consist of three fatty acids bonded to a glycerol molecule. Elevated blood triglyceride levels, like blood cholesterol levels, increase the risk of cardiovascular disease. Normal values for triglycerides fall between 50 to 150 milligrams per 100 milliliters of blood.

Unsaturated fats: Fats that contain double bonds between some of their carbon atoms. These double-bond positions are very vulnerable to attack by oxygen and free radicals.

Urea cycle: The metabolic process in which two molecules of ammonia are bonded to form the waste product urea. Urea is the final product of protein metabolism in humans.

Vasodilator: A substance that increases blood flow.

Vitamin A: One of the fat-soluble vitamins and an important antioxidant. Also called retinol, it is the form of vitamin A that is found in animals. It is essential to growth, healthy skin and epithelial tissue, and the prevention of night blindness.

Vitamin B_1 (thiamin): A member of the B-complex of vitamins that is essential for the health of brain and nerve tissue.

Vitamin B_2 (riboflavin): A member of the B-complex of vitamins that functions as an antioxidant cofactor, taking part in metabolic reactions involving proteins, fats, and carbohydrates.

Vitamin B₃ (niacinamide): A member of the B-complex of vitamins that is a particularly important coenzyme in the brain and nerve tissues. It is necessary for the synthesis of DNA, enhances the action of vitamin C and several amino acids, and is required for building the walls of brain cells.

Vitamin B₅ (pantothenic acid): A member of the B-complex of vitamins that acts as an antioxidant. It is also required for the conversion of choline to the neurotransmitter acetylcholine.

Vitamin B₆ (pyridoxine): A member of the B-complex of vitamins that acts as an antioxidant. It is necessary for the synthesis of DNA, enhancing the action of vitamin C and amino acids in the body and in their conversion into neurotransmitters in the brain.

Vitamin B₁₂ (cobalamin): A member of the B-complex of vitamins that is particularly important in the brain and nerve tissues.

Vitamin C: One of the most important antioxidant nutrients. Also called ascorbic acid, it is essential in building strong, healthy connective tissue.

Vitamin E: A fat-soluble, antioxidant vitamin chemically known as d-alpha-tocopherol.

VO₂ max: The maximum rate at which oxygen can be consumed—a measure of endurance fitness.

Zinc: A mineral found in substantial concentrations in the brain. It is a necessary factor in over twenty different enzymatic reactions and is essential for the production of the antioxidant enzyme SOD.

EAT TO WIN SOFTWARE FOR WINDOWS

If you own or have access to a personal computer, you can use the Eat to Win software program (for Windows 3.1, Windows 95, Windows 98 and higher, or Windows NT 3.51 or higher) to create Ultimate Ratio meals and recipes based on your favorite foods, drinks, spices, and fast foods. You can use it to analyze and construct diets for your family that conform to the Ultimate Ratio fat-loss and weight-maintenance plans.

The Eat to Win program contains the latest information on the nutritional content of hundreds of commonly eaten foods. The program also creates color pie charts of the ratios of protein, fat, and carbohydrate in your meals, recipes, and total daily diets. In addition, it enables you to graph the amino acid profiles of each food, recipe, and meal, as well as let you see the total nutrition breakdown of each. The program converts measures of weight and volume in a mouse click (e.g., grams to ounces, liquid volume to ounces, pounds to kilograms, tablespoons to grams or ounces, etc.). You can also modify recipes to create a new number of servings (the amounts of all ingredients are adjusted automatically), and you can save daily diets that you construct or new recipes to be recalled at a later time. The Eat to Win program lets you make "what if" changes to food quantities and see the nutritional effects of such changes in recipes and menus. You can also graph your progress to see how you are improving over time. No other nutritional software currently sold contains this information or these utilities. All of the recipes in this book were analyzed using the Eat to Win computer software program.

Programs like this one ordinarily cost hundreds of dollars, but for my readers the program is just $39.95 (this includes U.S. shipping and handling charges). If you would like a copy of this program, please send a check or money order to:

Small Planet Systems Corp.
P.O. Box 14-4272
Coral Gables, FL 33114-4272
Florida residents add $2.40 sales tax
Foreign orders add $10.00 for shipping and handling
For credit card orders, phone (305) 443-6011.

YOUR FIVE VITAL VALUES

When I introduced the concept of having an inexpensive blood chemistry test (called a blood chemistry profile) in my original book, *Eat to Win,* many people had never heard of their five vital values. Testing your blood for these values can tell you a lot about your current state of health and your risk of developing a serious health problem. I strongly recommend that you get a simple blood chemistry profile by visiting your doctor or a walk-in health-testing laboratory. Be sure to take the blood test after an overnight fast in order to obtain accurate values. Here are the five vital values you need to know (values are typically reported as mg %):

Total Cholesterol. Although many physicians believe that blood cholesterol levels are unimportant, the truth is that healthy individuals with sustained cholesterol levels of 150 mg % and below enjoy clean arteries. There are a number of issues that cloud the importance of keeping blood cholesterol levels at this optimum level, such as lipoprotein particle size (the protein-fat containers in which the body packages cholesterol for transport through the blood) and LDL/HDL-cholesterol ratios. You don't need to be concerned with these technical issues if you keep your total blood cholesterol level at 150 or below. If you want to avoid impotence, senility, hearing and vision loss, and coronary artery disease, do yourself a favor: Eat according to the Ultimate Ratio and drink a daily soy shake such as the *Purple Cow*—your cholesterol should settle nicely in the 150 range. A typically healthy range for total cholesterol is between 110 and 150.

HDL Cholesterol. Most people know this as the "good" cholesterol because it is associated with a decreased risk of heart disease. Moreover, people with HDL cholesterol levels of 70 mg % and above generally live into the ninth decade of life. A number of lifestyle choices affect HDL levels. Exercise and alcohol consumption tend to raise HDL levels, while high-fat diets, high-sugar consumption, and inactivity tend to cause lower HDL levels. On the Ultimate Ratio, as your total cholesterol drops, your HDL-cholesterol level (part of the total cholesterol number) may initially drop, then rise. As long as your total cholesterol number is at 150 mg % or below, it doesn't matter if you have a low HDL-cholesterol number (most likely, your physician is unaware of this). That's because at 150, there's not enough of the toxic form of cholesterol coursing through your circulatory system to cause heart disease. If you keep your cholesterol at 150 or below, your HDL value will probably settle between 30 and 70.

Triglycerides. "Triglycerides" is another name for fat. When you eat a meal, your liver responds by repackaging dietary fat into triglyceride molecules that then travel through the circulatory system to be stored as body fat or used in building the cell membranes. Elevated triglycerides are a risk factor for heart disease and other health problems, so you want to keep them as low as possible. Alcohol, sugar, dietary fat, and lack of exercise can all raise your triglyceride level. A healthy range for triglycerides is between 60 to 90.

Glucose. Also known as blood sugar, glucose in the blood is derived from dietary simple and complex carbohydrates and amino acids from muscle that the liver has converted to sugar. Diabetes is a condition characterized by an abnormally high blood sugar level (usually above 115 mg %) and hypoglycemia is a condition of abnormally low blood sugar (usually below 50). A typically healthy range for blood glucose is between 60 and 90.

Uric acid. Uric acid is a byproduct of nucleic acid metabolism. High uric acid levels can cause gout, a form of arthritis, and may increase the risk of cardiovascular disease. A typically healthy value for men is 4.0–6.5; women, 3.0–5.5.

I recommend having a blood chemistry profile done just before you begin the Ultimate Ratio and then four to six weeks later. If you are like most people, you will see a dramatic shift in your five vital values toward a healthier and more youthful set of values. This is your scientific proof that the Ultimate Ratio is working to make you healthier and fitter than ever before.

PRODUCT MANUFACTURERS LIST

Arizona
(Diet Green Tea with Ginseng, Diet Tea
   With Lemon)
Ferolito, Vultaggio & Sons
Lake Success, NY 11042
1-800-TEA-3775

Bertolli
(Extra Light Olive Oil)
Bertolli U.S.A. Inc.
Secaucus, NJ 07094
1-800-908-9789
www.bertolli.com

Boca Burger
(Boca Breakfast Links and Patties, Boca
   Burgers, Ground Boca Burger
   Recipe Basics)
www.bocaburger.com
Corporate Headquarters
20 N. Wacker Drive
Suite 1360
Chicago, IL 60606
312-201-0300

Borden
(Fat Free American Singles)
1-800-337-2407
cheese@bordenfoods.com

Bush's
(Chili Magic)
Bush Brothers & Company
P.O. Box 52330, Dept. C
Knoxville, TN 37950-2330

Carnation
(Malted Milk)
Nestlé USA
Beverage Division, Inc.
Glendale, CA 91203
1-800-673-8538

Classico
(Pecorino Romano and Herb Pasta
   Sauce, Roasted Peppers and Onions
   Pasta Sauce)
1-800-727-8260

International Gourmet Specialties
Company
180 East Broad Street
Columbus, OH 43215
e-mail: letters@classico.com

Dannon
(Vanilla Flavored Low Fat Yogurt)
The Dannon Company, Inc.
P.O. Box 1102
Maple Plain, MN 55592
1-800-321-2174

Del Monte
(Fresh Cut Diced Tomatoes; No Salt
Added)
Del Monte Foods
San Francisco, CA 94105
1-800-543-3090

Eagle Brand
(Fat Free Sweetened Condensed Milk)
Borden Foods
Columbus, OH 43215-3799

Egg Beaters
(Real Egg Substitute)
Nabisco
East Hanover, NJ 07936
1-800-NABISCO (622-4726)

Edensoy
(Original Soy Beverage)
Eden Foods, Inc.
701 Tecumseh Road
Clinton, MI 49236

French's
(Honey Mustard)
Reckitt & Colman, Inc.
Wayne, NJ 07474
1-800-841-1256

Green Giant
(Select, Baby Sweet Peas, Sugar Snap
Peas, Broccoli Florets, and Extra
Sweet Niblets Corn)

The Pillsbury Company
2866 Pillsbury Center
Minneapolis, MN 55402-1464
1-800-998-9996
www.greengiant.com

Health Valley
(Mild Vegetarian Chili With Lentils)
Health Valley Company, Inc.
16100 Foothill Blvd.
Irwindale, CA 91706-7811

Healthy Choice
(Low Fat Cheddar Cheese Natural
Fancy Shreds)
ConAgra Consumer Affairs
Dept. BC.
P.O. Box 3768
Omaha, NE 68103-0768
1-800-323-9980
www.healthychoice.com

Heinz
(Tomato Ketchup, Vegetarian Beans,
Sweet Relish)
(412) 456-5700
H. J. Heinz Co.
General Office
1062 Progress Street
Pittsburgh, PA 15212

Hershey's
(Genuine Chocolate Flavor Lite Syrup)
Hershey Chocolate USA
Hershey, PA 17035-0815
1-800-468-1714

Hunt's
(Manwich Sauce)
Hunt-Wesson, Inc.
P.O. Box 4800
Fullerton, CA 92834

Jell-O
(Cook and Serve Vanilla Flavor
Pudding and Pie Filling)
Kraft Foods, Inc.

Box JPPS-V
White Plains, NY 10625
1-800-431-1001

Kellogg's
(Just Right Fruit & Nut) Cereal
Kellogg
P.O. Box CAMB
Battle Creek, MI 49016
1-800-962-1413
www.Kelloggs.com

Kraft
(Macaroni and Cheese Dinner—
Original and Cheesy Alfredo) Easy
Mac, Whipped Cream Cheese, Light
Done Right salad dressings, and
Kraft Free salad dressings)
Kraft Foods, Inc.
www.kraftfoods.com
Glenview, IL 60025

Land O' Lakes
(Light Whipped Butter)
Arden Hills, MN 55126
1-800-328-4155

Lender's
Lender's Bagel Bakery
P.O. Box CAMB
Battle Creek, MI 49016-1986
1-800-432-3102

Lightlife
(Smart Deli Meatless Country Ham
Style Slices, Smart Deli Meatless
Roast Turkey Style Slices, Smart
Dogs)
P.O. Box 870
Greenfield, MA 01302
1-800-274-6001, Ext. 114
www.lightlife.com

Minute Maid
(100% Pure Lemon Juice)
Minute Maid Company
Division of The Coca-Cola Company

Houston, TX 77252
1-800-888-6488

Morningstar Farms
(Breakfast Patties, Breakfast Strips,
Chik Nuggets, Chik Patties, Veggie
Dogs, Harvest Burgers)
Worthington Foods
Worthington, OH 43085
1-614-885-9511

Nasoya
(Nayonaise)
1-800-229-8639
Distributed by Nasoya Foods, Inc.
Ayer, MA 01432

Ocean Spray
(Lightstyle Cranberry Juice Drink,
Lightstyle Cran-Mango Juice Drink,
Lightstyle Cran-Grape Juice Drink,
Lightstyle Cran-Raspberry Juice
Drink)
1-800-662-3263
Distributed by Ocean Spray
Cranberries, Inc.
A Grower Cooperative
Lakeville-Middleboro, MA 02349

Quaker
(Old Fashioned Oats, Instant
Oatmeal)
The Quaker Oats Company
P.O. Box 049003
Chicago, IL 60604-9003
1-800-555-OATS

Ragu
(Pizza Sauce)
Lipton
Englewood Cliffs, NJ 07632
1-800-328-7248
e-mail: letters@ragu.com

Ready Whip
(Fat Free Dairy Whipped Topping)
Beatrice Foods, Inc.

Waukesha, WI 53186
1-800-745-4514

Sargento
(Shredded Light Italian Cheese Blend,
   Light Deli Style Swiss Reduced Fat
   Cheese)
One Persnickety Place
Plymouth, WI 53073
1-800-CHEESES
www.sargento.com

Simply Potatoes
New Potato Wedges
Northern Star Company
3171 Fifth Street S.E.
Minneapolis, MN 55414

Soyco
(Lite and Less Veggy Parmesan Cheese
   Alternative)
Soyco Foods
2441 Viscount Row
Orlando, FL 32809
1-407-855-6600

Success
(10 Minute Brown Rice Boil in Bags)
Riviana Kitchens
P.O. Box 2636
Houston, TX 77252
1-800-226-9522
www.successrice.com

Swiss Miss
(Hot Cocoa Mix)
Hunt-Wesson, Inc.
P.O. Box 4800
Fullerton, CA 92834

Taco Bell
(Home Originals Fat Free Refried Beans)
Distributor: Kraft Foods, Inc.
Glenview, IL 60025
1-800-695-TACO

Thomas'
(Oat Bran English Muffins)
S.B. Thomas
General Offices
P.O. Box 535
Totowa, NJ 07511-0535

Twin Laboratories
(Choline Cocktail, Endurance Quick
   Fix, MaxiLIFE Soy Cocktail,
   MaxiLIFE Phytonutrient Cocktail)
150 Motor Parkway
Hauppauge, NY 11788
1-800-645-5626

V-8
(Spicy Hot Vegetable Juice)
Campbell Soup Company
Campbell Place
Camden, NJ 08103-1701

Westbrae Natural
(Westsoy Non Dairy Beverage 1% Lite)
1-800-SOY-MILK
www.westbrae.com

Yves Veggie Cuisine, Inc.
(Veggie Breakfast Links, Canadian
   Veggie Bacon, Veggie Deli Slices,
   Veggie Ground Round [Italian and
   Regular], Veggie Pepperoni, Veggie
   Pizza Pepperoni)
Delta (Vancouver), BC
Canada V3M 6R9

BIBLIOGRAPHY

Abbott WG, Swinburn B, Ruotolo G, et al. Effect of a high-carbohydrate, low-saturated-fat diet on apolipoprotein B and triglyceride metabolism in Pima Indians. *J Clin Invest,* 86:642–50, 1990 Aug.

Abernethy PJ, Thayer R, Taylor AW. Acute and chronic responses of skeletal muscle to endurance and sprint exercise. A review. *Sports Med,* 10:365–89, 1990 Dec.

Acheson KJ, Schutz Y, Bessard T, Anantharaman K, Flatt JP, Jequier E. Glycogen storage capacity and de novo lipogenesis during massive carbohydrate overfeeding in man. *Am J Clin Nutr,* 48:240–7, 1988 Aug.

Acheson KJ, Schutz Y, Bessard T, Flatt JP, Jequier E. Carbohydrate metabolism and de novo lipogenesis in human obesity. *Am J Clin Nutr,* 45:78–85, 1987 Jan.

Acheson KJ, Flatt JP, Jequier E. Glycogen synthesis versus lipogenesis after a 500 gram carbohydrate meal in man. *Metabolism,* 31:1234–40, 1982 Dec.

Ackerman NR, Arner EC, Galbraith W, Harris RR, Jaffee BD, Mackin WM. Anti-inflammatory consequences of 5-lipoxygenase inhibition. *Adv Prostaglandin Thromboxane Leukot Res,* 16:47–62, 1986.

Ackroff K, Sclafani A. Effects of the lipase inhibitor orlistat on intake and preference for dietary fat in rats. *Am J Physiol,* 271:R48–54, 1996 Jul.

Adam O. Anti-inflammatory diet in rheumatic diseases. *Eur J Clin Nutr,* 49:703–17, 1995 Oct.

Adams SO, Grady KE, Wolk CH, Mukaida C. Weight loss: a comparison of group and individual interventions. *J Am Diet Assoc,* 86:485–90, 1986 Apr.

Adembri C, Formigli L, Domenici Lobmardo L, Brunelleschi S, Novelli GP. [Effect of acetyl-carnitine in a model of muscle ischemia-reperfusion in humans.] *Minerva Anestesiol,* 57:1018–19, 1991 Oct.

Adibi S. Metabolism of branch-chain amino acids. *Metabolism,* 25(11):1287–1302, 1976.

Adlercreutz H, Markkanen H, Watanabe S. Plasma concentrations of phyto-oestrogens in Japanese men. *Lancet,* 342:1209–10, 1993.

Albert CM, Hennekens CH, CJ OD, et al. Fish consumption and risk of sudden cardiac death [see comments]. *JAMA,* 279:23–8, 1998 Jan 7.

Albertazzi P, Pansini F, Bonaccorsi G, Zanotti L, Forini E, De Aloysio D. The effect of dietary soy supplementation on hot flushes. *Obstet Gynecol,* 91:6–11, 1998 Jan.

Alford BB, Blankenship AC, Hagen RD. The effects of variations in carbohydrate, protein, and fat content of the diet upon weight loss, blood values, and nutrient intake of adult obese women. *J Am Diet Assoc,* 90:534–40, 1990 Apr.

Anderson JJ, Rondano P, Holmes A. Roles of diet and physical activity in the prevention of osteoporosis. *Scand J Rheumatol Suppl,* 103:65–74, 1996.

Andersson SO, Wolk A, Bergstrom R, Giovannucci E, Lindgren C. Energy, nutrient intake and prostate cancer risk: a population-based case-control study in Sweden. *Int J Cancer,* 68:716–22, 1996.

Anthony MS, Clarkson TB, Hughes CL, Jr., Morgan TM, Burke GL. Soybean isoflavones improve cardiovascular risk factors without affecting the reproductive system of peripubertal rhesus monkeys. *J Nutr,* 126:43–50, 1996.

Anton-Kuchly B, Ranganathan S, Potiron M, et al. Effect of a protein-sparing diet on responses to exercise in obese subjects. *J Sports Med Phys Fitness,* 33:59–64, 1993 Mar.

Aravanis C, Mensink RP, Karalias N, Christodoulou B, Kafatos A, Katan MB. Serum lipids, apoproteins and nutrient intake in rural Cretan boys consuming high-olive-oil diets. *J Clin Epidemiol,* 41:117–23, 1988.

Arenas J, Ricoy JR, Encinas AR, et al. Carnitine in muscle, serum, and urine of nonprofessional athletes: effects of physical exercise, training, and L-carnitine administration. *Muscle Nerve,* 14:598–604, 1991 Jul.

Arenas J, Huertas R, Campos Y, AE Di, Villalón JM, Vilas E. Effects of L-carnitine on the pyruvate dehydrogenase complex and carnitine palmitoyl transferase activities in muscle of endurance athletes. *FEBS Lett,* 341:91–3, 1994 Mar 14.

Ashutosh K, Methrotra K, Fragale-Jackson J. Effects of sustained weight loss and exercise on aerobic fitness in obese women. *J Sports Med Phys Fitness,* 37:252–7, 1997 Dec.

Assmann G, de Backer G, Bagnara S, et al. International consensus statement on olive oil and the Mediterranean diet: implications for health in Europe. The Olive Oil and the Mediterranean Diet Panel. *Eur J Cancer Prev,* 6:418–21, 1997 Oct.

Assmann G, de Backer G, Bagnara S, et al. Olive oil and the Mediterranean diet: implications for health in Europe. *Br J Nurs,* 6:675–7, 1997 June 26–Jul 9.

Atkinson G, Reilly T. Effects of age and time of day on preferred work rates during prolonged exercise. *Chronobiol Int,* 12:121–34, 1995 Apr.

Austen KF. The role of arachidonic acid metabolites in local and systemic inflammatory processes. *Drugs,* 33 Suppl 1:10–17, 1987.

Baekey PA, Cerda JJ, Burgin CW, Robbins FL, Rice RW, Baumgartner TG. Grapefruit pectin inhibits hypercholesterolemia and atherosclerosis in miniature swine. *Clin Cardiol,* 11:597–600, 1988.

Baggio G, Pagnan A, Muraca M, et al. Olive-oil-enriched diet: effect on serum lipoprotein levels and biliary cholesterol saturation. *Am J Clin Nutr,* 47:960–4, 1988 Jun.

Bangsbo J, Graham TE, Kiens B, Saltin B. Elevated muscle glycogen and anaerobic energy production during exhaustive exercise in man. *J Physiol* (Lond), 451:205–27, 1992.

Bangsbo J, Madsen K, Kiens B, Richter EA. Muscle glycogen synthesis in recovery from intense exercise in humans. *Am J Physiol,* 273:E416–24, 1997 Aug.

Barnes S, Peterson TG, Coward L. Rationale for the use of genistein-containing soy matrices in chemoprevention trials for breast and prostate cancer. *J Cell Biochem Suppl,* 22:181–7, 1995.

Barrett-Connor E, Friedlander NJ. Dietary fat, calories, and the risk of breast cancer in postmenopausal women: a prospective population-based study. *J Am Coll Nutr,* 12:390–9, 1993.

Barth CA, Behnke U. [Nutritional physiology of whey and whey components.] *Nahrung,* 41:2–12, 1997 Feb.

Beck SA, Smith KL, Tisdale MJ. Anticachectic and antitumor effect of eicosapentaenoic acid and its effect on protein turnover. *Cancer Res,* 51:6089–93, 1991.

Becker FF. Inhibition of spontaneous hepatocarcinogenesis in C3H/HeN mice by Edi Pro A, an isolated soy protein. *Carcinogenesis,* 2:1213–14, 1981.

Bell JD, Margen S, Calloway DH. Ketosis, weight loss, uric acid, and nitrogen balance in obese women fed single nutrients at low caloric levels. *Metabolism,* 18:193–208, 1969 Mar.

Bellush LL, Rowland N. Preference for high carbohydrate over various high fat diets by diabetic rats. *Physiol Behav,* 35:319–27, 1985 Sep.

Bemben MG. Age-related alterations in muscular endurance. *Sports Med,* 25:259–69, 1998 Apr.

Ben G, Gnudi L, Maran A., et al. Effects of chronic alcohol intake on carbohydrate and lipid metabolism in subjects with type II (non-insulin-dependent) diabetes. *Am J Med,* 90:70–6, 1991 Jan.

Berry EM, Eisenberg S, Friedlander Y, et al. Effects of diets rich in monounsaturated fatty acids on plasma lipoproteins—the Jerusalem Nutrition Study. II. Monounsaturated fatty acids vs carbohydrates. *Am J Clin Nutr,* 56:394–403, 1992 Aug.

Binkley NC, Suttie JW. Vitamin K nutrition and osteoporosis. *J Nutr,* 125:1812–21, 1995 Jul.

Birch LL. Children's preferences for high-fat foods. *Nutr Rev,* 50:249–55, 1992 Sep.

Birt DF, Pelling JC, Nair S, Lepley D. Diet intervention for modifying cancer risk. *Prog Clin Biol Res,* 395:223–34, 1996.

Bonjour JP, Schürch MA, Rizzoli R. Proteins and bone health. *Pathol Biol* (Paris), 45:57–9, 1997 Jan.

Bonjour JP, Schurch MA, Rizzoli R. Nutritional aspects of hip fractures. *Bone*, 18:S139–44, 1996 Mar.

Bosaeus I, Belfrage L, Lindgren C, Andersson H. Olive oil instead of butter increases net cholesterol excretion from the small bowel. *Eur J Clin Nutr*, 46:111–15, 1992 Feb.

Bougnoux P, Koscielny S, Chajès V, Deschamps P, Couet C, Calais G. Alpha-linolenic acid content of adipose breast tissue: a host determinant of the risk of early metastasis in breast cancer. *Br J Cancer*, 70:330–4, 1994.

Boutron MC, Faivre J, Marteau P, Couillault C, Senesse P, Quipourt V. Calcium, phosphorus, vitamin D, dairy products and colorectal carcinogenesis: a French case-control study. *Br J Cancer*, 74:145–51, 1996.

Bowtell JL, Gelly K, Jackman MI, Pate IA, Simeoni M, Rennie MJ. Effect of oral glutamine on whole body carbohydrate storage during recovery from exhaustive exercise. *J Applied Physiol*, 86:1770–7, 1999.

Boza J, Jiménez J, Baró L, Martínez O, Suárez MD, Gil A. Effects of native and hydrolyzed whey protein on intestinal repair of severely starved rats at weaning. *J Pediatr Gastroenterol Nutr*, 22:186–93, 1996 Feb.

Braga C, La Vecchia C, Franceschi S, et al. Olive oil, other seasoning fats, and the risk of colorectal carcinoma. *Cancer*, 82:448–53, 1998 Feb 1.

Brandi ML. Natural and synthetic isoflavones in the prevention and treatment of chronic diseases. *Calcif Tissue Int*, 61 Suppl 1:S5–8, 1997.

Brass EP, Hiatt WR. Carnitine metabolism during exercise. *Life Sci*, 54:1383–93, 1994.

Brass EP, Hiatt WR. The role of carnitine and carnitine supplementation during exercise in man and in individuals with special needs [see comments]. *J Am Coll Nutr*, 17:207–15, 1998 Jun.

Bruinoff TW, Brouwer CB, van Linde-Sibenius Trip M, Jansen H, Erkelens DW. Different postprandial metabolism of olive oil and soybean oil: a possible mechanism of the high-density lipoprotein conserving effect of olive oil. *Am J Clin Nutr*, 58:477–83, 1993 Oct.

Bunker VW. The role of nutrition in osteoporosis. *Br J Biomed Sci*, 51:228–40, 1994 Sep.

Burstein R, Prentice AM, Goldberg GR, Murgatroyd PR, Harding M, Coward WA. Metabolic fuel utilisation in obese women before and after weight loss. *Int J Obes Relat Metab Disord*, 20:253–9, 1996 Mar.

Burton GW TM, Acuff RV, et al. Human plasma and tissue alpha-tocopherol concentrations in response to supplementation with deuterated natural and synthetic vitamin E. *Am J Clin Nutr*, 67:669–84, 1998.

Cai Q, Wei H. Effect of dietary genistein on antioxidant enzyme activities in SENCAR mice. *Nutr Cancer*, 25:1–7, 1996.

Canalis E. Insulin-like growth factors and osteoporosis [comment]. *Bone*, 21:215–16, 1997 Sep.

Caputo FA, Mattes RD. Human dietary responses to perceived manipulation of fat content in a midday meal. *Int J Obes Relat Metab Disord*, 17:237–40, 1993 Apr.

Carabaza A, Ricart MD, Mor A, Guinovart JJ, Ciudad CJ. Role of AMP on the activation of glycogen synthase and phosphorylase by adenosine, fructose, and glutamine in rat hepatocytes. *J Biol Chem,* 265:2724–32, 1990 Feb 15.

Carreau JP, Lapous D, Raulin J. [A possible essential metabolite of linoleic acid: lipoic acid, the universal coenzyme of alpha-keto acid oxidation.] *C R Acad Sci Hebd Seances Acad Sci D,* 281:941–4, 1975 Sep 29.

Carroll KK, Jacobson EA, Eckel LA, Newmark HL. Calcium and carcinogenesis of the mammary gland. *Am J Clin Nutr,* 54:S206–8, 1991.

Catlett JP. Ketotic hypoglycemia. *W V Med J,* 79:126–8, 1983 Jun.

Cerretelli P, Marconi C. L-carnitine supplementation in humans. The effects on physical performance. *Int J Sports Med,* 11:1–14, 1990 Feb.

Chajès V, Sattler W, Stranzl A, Kostner GM. Influence of n-3 fatty acids on the growth of human breast cancer cells in vitro: relationship to peroxides and vitamin-E. *Breast Cancer Res Treat,* 34:199–212, 1995.

Chandler TJ. Physiology of aerobic fitness/endurance. *Instr Course Lect,* 43:11–15, 1994.

Chaudry A, McClinton S, Moffat LE, Wahle KW. Essential fatty acid distribution in the plasma and tissue phospholipids of patients with benign and malignant prostatic disease. *Br J Cancer,* 64:1157–60, 1991.

Chaudry AA, Wahle KW, McClinton S, Moffat LE. Arachidonic acid metabolism in benign and malignant prostatic tissue in vitro: effects of fatty acids and cyclooxygenase inhibitors. *Int J Cancer,* 57:176–80, 1994.

Chen C, Williams PF, Cooney GJ, Caterson ID, Turtle JR. The effects of fasting and refeeding on liver glycogen synthase and phosphorylase in obese and lean mice. *Horm Metab Res,* 24:161–6, 1992 Apr.

Clarkson PM. Nutritional ergogenic aids: carnitine. *Int J Sport Nutr,* 2:185–90, 1992 Jun.

Coggan AR, Spina RJ, Kohrt WM, Holloszy JO. Effect of prolonged exercise on muscle citrate concentration before and after endurance training in men. *Am J Physiol,* 264:E215–20, 1993 Feb.

Colditz GA, Willett WC, Stampfer MJ, et al. Weight as a risk factor for clinical diabetes in women. *Am J Epidemiol,* 132:501–13, 1990 Sep.

Conlay LA, Zeisel SH. Neurotransmitter precursors and brain function. *Neurosurgery,* 10:524–9, 1982 Apr.

Conlee RK, Hammer RL, Winder WW, Bracken ML, Nelson AG, Barnett DW. Glycogen repletion and exercise endurance in rats adapted to a high fat diet. *Metabolism,* 39:289–94, 1990 Mar.

Constantin-Teodosiu D, Howell S, Greenhaff PL. Carnitine metabolism in human muscle fiber types during submaximal dynamic exercise. *J Appl Physiol,* 80:1061–4, 1996 Mar.

Cook CB, Shawar L, Thompson H, Prasad C. Caloric intake and weight gain of rats depends on endogenous fat preference. *Physiol Behav,* 61:743–8, 1997 May.

Cooper C, Atkinson EJ, Hensrud DD, et al. Dietary protein intake and bone mass in women. *Calcif Tissue Int,* 58:320–5, 1996 May.

Cumming RG, Cummings SR, Nevitt MC, et al. Calcium intake and fracture risk: results from the study of osteoporotic fractures. *Am J Epidemiol,* 145:926–34, 1997 May 15.

Daily JWr, Sachan DS. Choline supplementation alters carnitine homeostasis in humans and guinea pigs. *J Nutr,* 125:1938–44, 1995 Jul.

Das UN. Gamma-linolenic acid, arachidonic acid, and eicosapentaenoic acid as potential anticancer drugs. *Nutrition,* 6:429–34, 1990.

Das UN. Free radicals: biology and relevance to disease. *J Assoc Physicians India,* 38:495–8, 1990.

Davies P, Bailey PJ, Goldenberg MM, Ford-Hutchinson AW. The role of arachidonic acid oxygenation products in pain and inflammation. *Annu Rev Immunol,* 2:335–57, 1984.

Davies P, Bonney RJ, Humes JL, Kuehl FA, Jr. Synthesis and release of oxygenation products of arachidonic acid by mononuclear phagocytes in response to inflammatory stimuli. *Inflammation,* 2:335–44, 1977 Dec.

Daviglus ML, Dyer AR, Persky V, et al. Dietary beta-carotene, vitamin C, and risk of prostate cancer: results from the Western Electric Study. *Epidemiology,* 7:472–7, 1996.

Deal CL. Osteoporosis: prevention, diagnosis, and management. *Am J Med,* 102:S35–9, 1997 Jan 27.

Decombaz J, Gmuender B, Sierro G, Cerretelli P. Muscle carnitine after strenuous endurance exercise. *J Appl Physiol,* 72:423–7, 1992 Feb.

Del Boca J, Flatt JP. Fatty acid synthesis from glucose and acetate and the control of lipogenesis in adipose tissue. *Eur J Biochem,* 11:127–34, 1969 Nov.

Dennis SC, Noakes TD, Hawley JA. Nutritional strategies to minimize fatigue during prolonged exercise: fluid, electrolyte and energy replacement. *J Sports Sci,* 15:305–13, 1997 Jun.

Dimitriadis E, Griffin M, Collins P, Johnson A, Owens D, Tomkin GH. Lipoprotein composition in NIDDM: effects of dietary oleic acid on the composition, oxidisability and function of low and high density lipoproteins. *Diabetologia,* 39(6):667–76, 1996.

Donnelly JE, Sharp T, Houmard J, et al. Muscle hypertrophy with large-scale weight loss and resistance training. *Am J Clin Nutr,* 58:561–5, 1993 Oct.

Dreher ML, Maher CV, Kearney P. The traditional and emerging role of nuts in healthful diets. *Nutr Rev,* 54:241–5, 1996 Aug.

Drewnowski A. Dietary fats: perceptions and preferences. *J Am Coll Nutr,* 9:431–5, 1990 Aug.

Drewnowski A. Sensory preferences for fat and sugar in adolescence and adult life. *Ann N Y Acad Sci,* 561:243–50, 1989.

Drewnowski A, Krahn DD, Demitrack MA, Nairn K, Gosnell BA. Taste responses and preferences for sweet high-fat foods: evidence for opioid involvement. *Physiol Behav,* 51:371–9, 1992 Feb.

Drewnowski A, Kurth C, Holden-Wiltse J, Saari J. Food preferences in human obesity: carbohydrates versus fats. *Appetite,* 18:207–21, 1992 Jun.

Drewnowski A, Greenwood MR. Cream and sugar: human preferences for high-fat foods. *Physiol Behav,* 30:629–33, 1983 Apr.

Drovanti A, Bignamini A, Rovati A. Therapeutic activity of oral glucosamine sulfate in osteoarthritis: a placebo-controlled double-blind investigation. *Clinical Therapeutics,* 3:260–72, 1999.

Dulloo AG. Human pattern of food intake and fuel-partitioning during weight recovery after starvation: a theory of autoregulation of body composition. *Proc Nutr Soc,* 56:25–40, 1997 Mar.

Dulloo AG, Geissler CA, Horton T, Collins A, Miller DS. Normal caffeine consumption: influence on thermogenesis and daily energy expenditure in lean and postobese human volunteers. *Am J Clin Nutr,* 49:44–50, 1989 Jan.

Dulloo AG, Girardier L. Adaptive changes in energy expenditure during refeeding following low-calorie intake: evidence for a specific metabolic component favoring fat storage. *Am J Clin Nutr,* 52:415–20, 1990 Sep.

Dulloo AG, Jacquet J, Girardier L. Poststarvation hyperphagia and body fat overshooting in humans: a role for feedback signals from lean and fat tissues. *Am J Clin Nutr,* 65:717–23, 1997 Mar.

Dulloo AG, Miller DS. Obesity: a disorder of the sympathetic nervous system. *World Rev Nutr Diet,* 50:1–56, 1987.

Dulloo AG, Jacquet J, Girardier L. Autoregulation of body composition during weight recovery in humans: the Minnesota Experiment revisited. *Int J Obes Relat Metab Disord,* 20:393–405, 1996 May.

Dulloo AG, Jacquet J. Adaptive reduction in basal metabolic rate in response to food deprivation in humans: a role for feedback signals from fat stores. *Am J Clin Nutr,* 68:599–606, 1998 Sep.

Dulloo AG, Mensi N, Seydoux J, Girardier L. Differential effects of high-fat diets varying in fatty acid composition on the efficiency of lean and fat tissue deposition during weight recovery after low food intake. *Metabolism,* 44:273–9, 1995 Feb.

Durlach J, et al. Magnesium and ageing. II. Clinical data: aetiological mechanisms and pathophysiological consequences of magnesium deficit in the elderly. *Magnes Res,* 6(4):379–94, 1993.

Dwyer JT, Goldin BR, Saul N, Gualtieri L, Barakat S, Adlercreutz H. Tofu and soy drinks contain phytoestrogens. *J Am Diet Assoc,* 94:739–43, 1994.

Dyck DJ, Peters SJ, Wendling PS, Chesley A, Hultman E, Spriet LL. Regulation of muscle glycogen phosphorylase activity during intense aerobic cycling with elevated FFA. *Am J Physiol,* 270:E116–25, 1996 Jan.

Eaton-Evans J. Osteoporosis and the role of diet. *Br J Biomed Sci,* 51:358–70, 1994 Dec.

Ebeling P, Tuominen JA, Arenas J, Garcia Benayas C, Koivisto VA. The association of acetyl-L-carnitine with glucose and lipid metabolism in human muscle in vivo: the effect of hyperinsulinemia. *Metabolism,* 46:1454–7, 1997 Dec.

Elizalde G, Sclafani A. Fat appetite in rats: flavor preferences conditioned by nutritive and non-nutritive oil emulsions. *Appetite,* 15:189–97, 1990 Dec.

Ells GW, Chisholm KA, Simmons VA, Horrobin DF. Vitamin E blocks the cyto-toxic effect of gamma-linolenic acid when administered as late as the time of onset of cell death—insight into the mechanism of fatty acid induced cytotoxic-ity. *Cancer Lett,* 98:207–11, 1996.

Engell D, Bordi P, Borja M, Lambert C, Rolls B. Effects of information about fat content on food preferences in pre-adolescent children. *Appetite,* 30:269–82, 1998 Jun.

Epstein LH, Wing RR, Penner BC, Kress MJ. Effect of diet and controlled exercise on weight loss in obese children. *J Pediatr,* 107:358–61, 1985 Sept.

Estrada DE, Ewart HS, Tsakiridis T, et al. Stimulation of glucose uptake by the nat-ural coenzyme alpha-lipoic acid/thioctic acid: participation of elements of the insulin signaling pathway. *Diabetes,* 45:1798–804, 1996 Dec.

Falconer JS, Ross JA, Fearon KC, Hawkins RA, MG OR, Carter DC. Effect of eicosapentaenoic acid and other fatty acids on the growth in vitro of human pan-creatic cancer cell lines. *Br J Cancer,* 69:826–32, 1994.

Felber JP, Haesler E, E Je. Metabolic origin of insulin resistance in obesity with and without type 2 (non-insulin-dependent) diabetes mellitus. *Diabetologia,* 36:1221–9, 1993 Dec.

Ferris SH, Sathananthan G, Reisberg B, Gershon S. Long-term choline treatment of memory-impaired elderly patients. *Science,* 205:1039–40, 1979 Sept 7.

Feskanich D, Willett WC, Stampfer MJ, Colditz GA. Milk, dietary calcium, and bone fractures in women: a 12-year prospective study. *Am J Public Health,* 87:992–7, 1997 Jun.

Feskanich D, Willett WC, Stampfer MJ, Colditz GA. Protein consumption and bone fractures in women. *Am J Epidemiol,* 143:472–9, 1996 Mar 1.

Feuerstein G, Hallenbeck JM. Leukotrienes in health and disease. *FASEB J,* 1:186–92, 1987 Sep.

Fiatarone MA, EF ON, Ryan ND, et al. Exercise training and nutritional supple-mentation for physical frailty in very elderly people [see comments]. *N Engl J Med,* 330:1769–75, 1994 Jun 23.

Fielding R. The role of progressive resistance training and nutrition in the preserva-tion of lean body mass in the elderly. *J Am Coll Nutr,* 14(6):587–94, 1995.

Fisher JO, Birch LL. Fat preferences and fat consumption of 3- to 5-year-old chil-dren are related to parental adiposity. *J Am Diet Assoc,* 95:759–64, 1995 Jul.

Fisher WE, Boros LG, Schirmer WJ. Reversal of enhanced pancreatic cancer growth in diabetes by insulin. *Surgery,* 118:453–7, 1995.

Flatt JP. Glycogen levels and obesity. *Int J Obes Relat Metab Disord,* 20 Suppl 2:S1–11, 1996 Mar.

Flatt JP. Carbohydrate balance and body-weight regulation. *Proc Nutr Soc,* 55:449–65, 1996 Mar.

Flatt JP. Body composition, respiratory quotient, and weight maintenance. *Am J Clin Nutr,* 62:S1107–17, 1995 Nov.

Flatt JP. Integration of the overall response to exercise. *Int J Obes Relat Metab Dis-ord,* 19 Suppl 4:S31–40, 1995 Oct.

Flatt JP. McCollum Award Lecture, 1995: diet, lifestyle, and weight maintenance. *Am J Clin Nutr,* 62:820–36, 1995 Oct.

Flatt JP. Carbohydrate balance and food intake regulation [letter; comment]. *Am J Clin Nutr,* 62:155–7, 1995 Jul.

Flatt JP. Use and storage of carbohydrate and fat. *Am J Clin Nutr,* 61:S952–9, 1995 Apr.

Flatt JP. The difference in the storage capacities for carbohydrate and for fat, and its implications in the regulation of body weight. *Ann N Y Acad Sci,* 499:104–23, 1987.

Flatt JP. Importance of nutrient balance in body weight regulation. *Diabetes Metab Rev,* 4:571–81, 1988 Sep.

Flatt JP. Dietary fat, carbohydrate balance, and weight maintenance: effects of exercise. *Am J Clin Nutr,* 45:296–306, 1987 Jan.

Flatt JP. Conversion of carbohydrate to fat in adipose tissue: an energy-yielding and, therefore, self-limiting process. *J Lipid Res,* 11:131–43, 1970 Mar.

Flatt JP, Ball EG. The role of reduced coenzymes and oxygen in the control of fatty acid synthesis in adipose tissue. *Biochem Soc Symp,* 24:75–7, 1963.

Flatt JP. Role of the increased adipose tissue mass in the apparent insulin insensitivity of obesity. *Am J Clin Nutr,* 25:1189–92, 1972 Nov.

Flatt JP. On the maximal possible rate of ketogenesis. *Diabetes,* 21:50–3, 1972 Jan.

Flatt JP. Energy metabolism and the control of lipogenesis in adipose tissue. *Horm Metab Res,* 2: Suppl 2:93–101, 1970.

Flatt JP. How NOT to approach the obesity problem. *Obes Res,* 5:632–3, 1997 Nov.

Fogelholm GM, Koskinen R, Laakso J, Rankinen T, Ruokonen I. Gradual and rapid weight loss: effects on nutrition and performance in male athletes. *Med Sci Sports Exerc,* 25:371–7, 1993 Mar.

Foreyt JP, Reeves RS, Darnell LS, Wohlleb JC, Gotto AM. Soup consumption as a behavioral weight loss strategy. *J Am Diet Assoc,* 86:524–6, 1986 Apr.

Foster GD, Wadden TA, Kendrick ZV, Letizia KA, Lander DP, Conill AM. The energy cost of walking before and after significant weight loss. *Med Sci Sports Exerc,* 27:888–94, 1995 Jun.

Franke AA, Custer LJ. Daidzein and genistein concentrations in human milk after soy consumption. *Clin Chem,* 42:955–64, 1996.

Freyssenet D, Berthon P, Denis C, Barthelemy JC, Guezennec CY, Chatard JC. Effect of a 6-week endurance training programme and branched-chain amino acid supplementation on histomorphometric characteristics of aged human muscle. *Arch Physiol Biochem,* 104:157–62, 1996.

Fried PI, McClean PA, Phillipson EA, Zamel N, Murray FT, Marliss EB. Effect of ketosis on respiratory sensitivity to carbon dioxide in obesity. *N Engl J Med,* 294:1081–6, 1976 May 13.

Friedewald WT, Thom TJ. Decline of coronary heart disease mortality in the United States. *Isr J Med Sci,* 22:307–12, 1986.

Friedman JE, Caro JF, Pories WJ, Azevedo JL, Jr., Dohm GL. Glucose metabolism in incubated human muscle: effect of obesity and non-insulin-dependent diabetes mellitus. *Metabolism,* 43:1047–54, 1994 Aug.

Friedmann B, Kindermann W. Energy metabolism and regulatory hormones in women and men during endurance exercise. *Eur J Appl Physiol,* 59:1–9, 1989.

Friolet R, Hoppeler H, Krähenbühl S. Relationship between the coenzyme A and the carnitine pools in human skeletal muscle at rest and after exhaustive exercise under normoxic and acutely hypoxic conditions. *J Clin Invest,* 94:1490–5, 1994 Oct.

Fritsché R, Pahud JJ, Pecquet S, Pfeifer A. Induction of systemic immunologic tolerance to beta-lactoglobulin by oral administration of a whey protein hydrolysate. *J Allergy Clin Immunol,* 100:266–73, 1997 Aug.

Fukagawa NK, Anderson JW, Hageman G, Young VR, Minaker KL. High-carbohydrate, high-fiber diets increase peripheral insulin sensitivity in healthy young and old adults. *Am J Clin Nutr,* 52:524–8, 1990 Sep.

Fukutake M, Takahashi M, Ishida K, Kawamura H, Sugimura T. Quantification of genistein and genistin in soybeans and soybean products. 1996.

Garland C, Shekelle RB, Barrett-Connor E, Criqui MH, Rossof AH, Paul O. Dietary vitamin D and calcium and risk of colorectal cancer: a 19-year prospective study in men. *Lancet,* 1:307–9, 1985.

Garriga J, Cussó R. Effect of starvation on glycogen and glucose metabolism in different areas of the rat brain. *Brain Res,* 591:277–82, 1992 Sept 25.

Garrow JS. Is body fat distribution changed by dieting? *Acta Med Scand Suppl,* 723:199–203, 1988.

Giamberardino MA, Dragani L, Valente R, Di Lisa F, Saggini R, Vecchiet L. Effects of prolonged L-carnitine administration on delayed muscle pain and CK release after eccentric effort. *Int J Sports Med,* 17:320–4, 1996 Jul.

Giovannucci E, Stampfer MJ, Colditz GA, Rimm EB, Trichopoulos D, Rosner BA. Folate, methionine, and alcohol intake and risk of colorectal adenoma. *J Natl Cancer Inst,* 85:875–84, 1993.

Giovannucci E, Rimm EB, Ascherio A, Stampfer MJ, Colditz GA, Willett WC. Alcohol, low-methionine, low-folate diets, and risk of colon cancer in men. *J Natl Cancer Inst,* 87:265–73, 1995.

Giovannucci E. How is individual risk for prostate cancer assessed? *Hematol Oncol Clin North Am,* 10:537–48, 1996.

Giovenali P, Fenocchio D, Montanari G, et al. Selective trophic effect of L-carnitine in type I and IIa skeletal muscle fibers. *Kidney Int,* 46:1616–19, 1994 Dec.

Goetzl EJ. Oxygenation products of arachidonic acid as mediators of hypersensitivity and inflammation. *Med Clin North Am,* 65:809–28, 1981 Jul.

Goforth HW, Jr., Arnall DA, Bennett BL, Law PG. Persistence of supercompensated muscle glycogen in trained subjects after carbohydrate loading. *J Appl Physiol,* 82:342–7, 1997 Jan.

Golay A, Felber JP. Evolution from obesity to diabetes. *Diabetes Metab,* 20:3–14, 1994 Jan.–Feb.

Goldstein MR. Nuts, nuts good for your heart . . . ? [letter; comment]. *Arch Intern Med,* 152:2507, 2511, 1992 Dec.

González ER. Studies show the obese may prefer fats to sweets [news]. *JAMA,* 250:579, 583, 1983 Aug 5.

Gooderham MH, Adlercreutz H, Ojala ST, K Wĺ, Holub BJ. A soy protein isolate rich in genistein and daidzein and its effects on plasma isoflavone concentrations, platelet aggregation, blood lipids and fatty acid composition of plasma phospholipids in normal men. *J Nutr,* 126:2000–6, 1996.

Grammatikos SI, Subbaiah PV, Victor TA, Miller WM. n-3 and n-6 fatty acid processing and growth effects in neoplastic and non-cancerous human mammary epithelial cell lines. *Br J Cancer,* 70:219–27, 1994.

Granström E. The arachidonic acid cascade. The prostaglandins, thromboxanes and leukotrienes. *Inflammation,* 8 Suppl:S15–25, 1984 Jun.

Greenhaff P. Renal dysfunction accompanying oral creatine supplements. *Lancet,* 352:233–4.

Grey NJ, Karl I, Kipnis DM. Physiologic mechanisms in the development of starvation ketosis in man. *Diabetes,* 24:10–16, 1975 Jan.

Griffiths AJ, Humphreys SM, Clark ML, Fielding BA, Frayn KN. Immediate metabolic availability of dietary fat in combination with carbohydrate. *Am J Clin Nutr,* 59:53–9, 1994 Jan.

Griffiths DE, Cain K, Hyams RL. Oxidative phosphorylation: a new biological function for lipoic acid. *Biochem Soc Trans,* 5:205–7, 1977.

Gwinup G. Weight loss without dietary restriction: efficacy of different forms of aerobic exercise. *Am J Sports Med,* 15:275–9, 1987 May–Jun.

Hackney AC. Endurance training and testosterone levels. *Sports Med,* 8:117–27, 1989 Aug.

Haenszel W, Kurihara M. Studies of Japanese migrants. I. Mortality from cancer and other diseases among Japanese in the United States. *J Natl Cancer Inst,* 40:43–68, 1968 Jan.

Hanai T, Hashimoto T, Nishiwaki K, et al. Comparison of prostanoids and their precursor fatty acids in human hepatocellular carcinoma and noncancerous reference tissues. *J Surg Res,* 54:57–60, 1993.

Hardin CD, Roberts TM. Differential regulation of glucose and glycogen metabolism in vascular smooth muscle by exogenous substrates. *J Mol Cell Cardiol,* 29:1207–16, 1997 Apr.

Hardman AE, Williams C, Wootton SA. The influence of short-term endurance training on maximum oxygen uptake, submaximum endurance and the ability to perform brief, maximal exercise. *J Sports Sci,* 4:109–16, 1986 Autumn.

Hardman AE, Williams C. Increased dietary carbohydrate and endurance during single-leg cycling using a limb with normal muscle glycogen concentration. *J Sports Sci,* 7:127–38, 1989 Summer.

Haskin CL, Milam SB, Cameron IL. Pathogenesis of degenerative joint disease in the human temporomandibular joint. *Crit Rev Oral Biol Med,* 6:248–77, 1995.

Hawrylewicz EJ, Zapata JJ, Blair WH. Soy and experimental cancer: animal studies. *J Nutr,* 125:S698–708, 1995.

Haymond MW, Howard C, Ben-Galim E, DeVivo DC. Effects of ketosis on glucose flux in children and adults. *Am J Physiol,* 245:E373–8, 1983 Oct.

Heaney RP. Pathophysiology of osteoporosis. *Am J Med Sci,* 312:251–6, 1996 Dec.

Heatherton TF, Polivy J, Herman CP. Restraint, weight loss, and variability of body weight. *J Abnorm Psychol,* 100:78–83, 1991 Feb.

Heber D, Ashley JM, Leaf DA, Barnard RJ. Reduction of serum estradiol in post-menopausal women given free access to low-fat high-carbohydrate diet. *Nutrition,* 7:137–9; discussion 139–40, 1991 Mar–Apr.

Heinonen OJ. Carnitine and physical exercise. *Sports Med,* 22:109–32, 1996 Aug.

Heller A, Koch T, Schmeck J, van Ackern K. Lipid mediators in inflammatory disorders. *Drugs,* 55:487–96, 1998 Apr.

Hendrich S, Lee KW, Xu X, Wang HJ, Murphy PA. Defining food components as new nutrients. *J Nutr,* 124:S1789–92, 1994.

Hersey WCr, Graves JE, Pollock ML, et al. Endurance exercise training improves body composition and plasma insulin responses in 70- to 79-year-old men and women. *Metabolism,* 43:847–54, 1994 Jul.

Hickner RC, Fisher JS, Hansen PA, et al. Muscle glycogen accumulation after endurance exercise in trained and untrained individuals. *J Appl Physiol,* 83:897–903, 1997 Sep.

Higashi K, Ishikawa T, Shige H, et al. Olive oil increases the magnitude of postprandial chylomicron remnants compared to milk fat and safflower oil. *J Am Coll Nutr,* 16:429–34, 1997 Oct.

Higgs GA. The role of eicosanoids in inflammation. *Prog Lipid Res,* 25:555–61, 1986.

Honn KV, Nelson KK, Renaud C, Bazaz R, Diglio CA, Timar J. Fatty acid modulation of tumor cell adhesion to microvessel endothelium and experimental metastasis. *J Prostaglandins,* 44:413–29, 1992.

Hopewell JW, Robbins ME, van den Aardweg GJ, Morris GM, Ross GA, Whitehouse. The modulation of tradition-induced damage to pig skin by essential fatty acids. *Br J Cancer,* 68:1–7, 1993.

Hoppel CL, Genuth SM. Urinary excretion of acetylcarnitine during human diabetic and fasting ketosis. *Am J Physiol,* 243:E168–72, 1982 Aug.

Houmard JA, Wheeler WS, McCammon MR, et al. An evaluation of waist to hip ratio measurement methods in relation to lipid and carbohydrate metabolism in men. *Int J Obes,* 15:181–8, 1991 Mar.

Houtkooper L. Food selection for endurance sports. *Med Sci Sports Exerc,* 24:S349–59, 1992 Sept.

Howard AN. The historical development, efficacy and safety of very-low-calorie diets. *Int J Obes,* 5:195–208, 1981.

Howell TJ, MacDougall DE, Jones PJ. Phytosterols partially explain differences in cholesterol metabolism caused by corn or olive oil feeding. *J Lipid Res,* 39:892–900, 1998 Apr.

Huang Z, Hankinson SE, Colditz GA, et al. Dual effects of weight and weight gain on breast cancer risk [see comments]. *JAMA,* 278:1407–11, 1997 Nov 5.

Huertas R, Campos Y, E Di, et al. Respiratory chain enzymes in muscle of endurance athletes: effect of L-carnitine. *Biochem Biophys Res Commun,* 188:102–7, 1992 Oct 15.

Hutchins AM, Slavin JL, Lampe JW. Urinary isoflavonoid phytoestrogen and lignan excretion after consumption of fermented and unfermented soy products. *J Am Diet Assoc,* 95:545–51, 1995.

Ivy JL, Lee MC, Brozinick JT, Jr., Reed MJ. Muscle glycogen storage after different amounts of carbohydrate ingestion. *J Appl Physiol,* 65:2018–23, 1988 Nov.

Jayanthi S, Jayanthi G, Varalakshmi P. Effect of DL–alpha-lipoic acid on some carbohydrate metabolising enzymes in stone forming rats. *Biochem Int,* 25:123–36, 1991 Sep.

Jenkins DJ, Popovich DG, Kendall CW, et al. Effect of a diet high in vegetables, fruit, and nuts on serum lipids. *Metabolism,* 46:530–7, 1997 May.

Jensen J, Aslesen R, Ivy JL, Brørs O. Role of glycogen concentration and epinephrine on glucose uptake in rat epitrochlearis muscle. *Am J Physiol,* 272:E649–55, 1997 Apr.

Jensen J, Oftebro H, Breigan B, et al. Comparison of changes in testosterone concentrations after strength and endurance exercise in well trained men. *Eur J Appl Physiol,* 63:467–71, 1991.

Jerusalinsky D, Kornisiuk E, Izquierdo I. Cholinergic neurotransmission and synaptic plasticity concerning memory processing. *Neurochem Res,* 22:507–15, 1997 Apr.

Jeukendrup AE, Saris WH, Wagenmakers AJ. Fat metabolism during exercise: a review. Part I: fatty acid mobilization and muscle metabolism. *Int J Sports Med,* 19:231–44, 1998 May.

Jiang WG, Hiscox S, Hallett MB, Horrobin DF, Mansel RE, Puntis MC. Regulation of the expression of E-cadherin on human cancer cells by gamma-linolenic acid (GLA). *Cancer Res,* 55:5043–8, 1995.

Johnson SL, McPhee L, Birch LL. Conditioned preferences: young children prefer flavors associated with high dietary fat. *Physiol Behav,* 50:1245–51, 1991 Dec.

Johnson RH, Walton JL. Fitness, fatness, and post-exercise ketosis. *Lancet,* 1:566–8, 1971 Mar 20.

Joossens JV, Geboers J. Nutrition and cancer. *Biomed Pharmacother,* 40:127–38, 1986.

Kagan A, Rhoads GG, Zeegen PD, Nichaman MZ. Coronary heart disease among men of Japanese ancestry in Hawaii. The Honolulu heart study. *Isr J Med Sci,* 7:1573–7, 1971 Dec.

Kanter MM, Williams MH. Antioxidants, carnitine, and choline as putative ergogenic aids. *Int J Sport Nutr,* 5 Suppl:S120–31, 1995 Jun.

Karhunen LJ, Lappalainen RI, Haffner SM, et al. Serum leptin, food intake and preferences for sugar and fat in obese women. *Int J Obes Relat Metab Disord,* 22:819–21, 1998 Aug.

Karmann H, Mrosovsky N, Heitz A, Le Maho Y. Protein sparing on very low calorie diets: ground squirrels succeed where obese people fail. *Int J Obes Relat Metab Disord,* 18:351–3, 1994 May.

Kennedy AR. The evidence for soybean products as cancer preventive agents. *J Nutr,* 125:S733–43, 1995.

Kern DL, McPhee L, Fisher J, Johnson S, Birch LL. The postingestive consequences of fat condition preferences for flavors associated with high dietary fat. *Physiol Behav,* 54:71–6, 1993 Jul.

Kida Y, Esposito-Del Puente A, Bogardus C, Mott DM. Insulin resistance is associated with reduced fasting and insulin-stimulated glycogen synthase phosphatase activity in human skeletal muscle. *J Clin Invest,* 85:476–81, 1990 Feb.

Kim JG, Lee JY. Serum insulin-like growth factor binding protein profiles in postmenopausal women: their correlation with bone mineral density. *Am J Obstet Gynecol,* 174:1511–7, 1996 May.

Kim YI, Mason JB. Nutrition chemoprevention of gastrointestinal cancers: a critical review. *Nutr Rev,* 54:259–79, 1996.

King RA, Broadbent JL, Head RJ. Absorption and excretion of the soy isoflavone genistein in rats. *J Nutr,* 126:176–82, 1996.

Kinscherf R, Hack V, Fischbach T, et al. Low plasma glutamine in combination with high glutamate levels indicate risk for loss of body cell mass in healthy individuals: the effect of N-acetyl-cysteine. *J Mol Med,* 74:393–400, 1996 Jul.

Kiritsakis A, Markakis P. Olive oil: a review. *Adv Food Res,* 31:453–82, 1987.

Klein RF. Alcohol-induced bone disease: impact of ethanol on osteoblast proliferation. *Alcohol Clin Exp Res,* 21:392–9, 1997 May.

Klein S, Wolfe RR. Carbohydrate restriction regulates the adaptive response to fasting. *Am J Physiol,* 262:E631–6, 1992 May.

Kohrt WM, Landt M, Birge SJ, Jr. Serum leptin levels are reduced in response to exercise training, but not hormone replacement therapy, in older women. *J Clin Endocrinol Metab,* 81:3980–5, 1996 Nov.

Kolonel LN. Nutrition and prostate cancer. *Cancer Causes Control,* 7:83–4, 1996.

Kolonel LN, Hankin JH, Nomura AM. Multiethnic studies of diet, nutrition, and cancer in Hawaii. *Princess Takamatsu Symp,* 16:29–40, 1985.

Kolonel LN, Hankin JH, Yoshizawa CN. Vitamin A and prostate cancer in elderly men: enhancement of risk. *Cancer Res,* 47:2982–5, 1987.

Konig W, Bremm KD, Brom HJ, et al. The role of leukotriene-inducing and -metabolizing enzymes in inflammation. *Int Arch Allergy Appl Immunol,* 82:526–31, 1987.

Krahn DD, Gosnell BA. Fat-preferring rats consume more alcohol than carbohydrate-preferring rats. *Alcohol,* 8:313–16, 1991 Jul–Aug.

Kreitzman SN, Coxon AY, Szaz KF. Glycogen storage: illusions of easy weight loss, excessive weight regain, and distortions in estimates of body composition. *Am J Clin Nutr,* 56:S292–3, 1992 Jul.

Kris-Etherton PM, Derr JA, Mustad VA, Seligson FH, Pearson TA. Effects of a milk chocolate bar per day substituted for a high-carbohydrate snack in young men on an NCEP/AHA Step 1 Diet. *Am J Clin Nutr,* 60:S1037–42, 1994 Dec.

Lamartiniere CA, Moore JB, Brown NM, Thompson R, Hardin MJ, Barnes S. Genistein suppresses mammary cancer in rats. *Carcinogenesis,* 16:2833–40, 1995.

Lands WE. Control of prostaglandin biosynthesis. *Prog Lipid Res,* 20:875–83, 1981.

Langfort J, Pilis W, Zarzeczny R, Nazar K, Kaciuba UsH. Effect of low-carbohydrate-ketogenic diet on metabolic and hormonal responses to graded exercise in men. *J Physiol Pharmacol,* 47:361–71, 1996 Jun.

Lauritsen K, Laursen LS, Bukhave K, Rask-Madsen J. Does vitamin E supplementation modulate in vivo arachidonate metabolism in human inflammation? *Pharmacol Toxicol,* 61:246–9, 1987 Oct.

la Vecchia C, Negri E. Franceschi S, Decarli A, Giacosa A, Lipworth L. Olive oil, other dietary fats, and the risk of breast cancer (Italy). *Cancer Causes Control,* 6:545–50, 1995 Nov.

Lavoie C, F Pe, Chiasson JL. Role of the sympathoadrenal system in the regulation of glycogen metabolism in resting and exercising skeletal muscles. *Horm Metab Res,* 24:266–71, 1992 Jun.

Lawrence JC, Jr., Roach PJ. New insights into the role and mechanism of glycogen synthase activation by insulin. *Diabetes,* 46:541–7, 1997 Apr.

Leaf A, Frisa, KB. Eating for health or for athletic performance? *Am J Clin Nutr,* 49:1066–9, 1989.

Lean ME, Han TS, Prvan T, Richmond PR, Avenell A. Weight loss with high and low carbohydrate 1200 kilocalorie diets in free-living women. *Eur J Clin Nutr,* 51:243–8, 1997 Apr.

Lee IM, Manson JE, Hennekens CH, Paffenbarger RS, Jr. Body weight and mortality. A 27-year follow-up of middle-aged men [see comments]. *JAMA,* 270:2823–8, 1993 Dec 15.

Leenen R, van der Kooy K, Seidell JC, Deurenberg P, Koppeschaar HP. Visceral fat accumulation in relation to sex hormones in obese men and women undergoing weight loss therapy. *J Clin Endocrinol Metab,* 78:1515–20, 1994 Jun.

Lefkowith JB, Klahr S. Polyunsaturated fatty acids and renal disease. *Proc Soc Exp Biol Med,* 213:13–23, 1996 Oct.

Leitzmann MF, Willett W, Rimm E, et al. A prospective study of coffee consumption and the risk of symptomatic gallstone disease in men. *JAMA,* 281:2106–12, 1999.

Leung LH. Pantothenic acid as a weight-reducing agent: fasting without hunger, weakness and ketosis. *Med Hypotheses,* 44:403–5, 1995 May.

Lewis GP. Biochemistry, pathophysiology and pharmacology of slow-reacting substances/leukotrienes. *Agents Actions,* 11:569–71, 1981 Dec.

Lewis RA, Austen KF. The biologically active leukotrienes. Biosynthesis, metabolism, receptors, functions, and pharmacology. *J Clin Invest,* 73:889–97, 1984 Apr.

Lewis RA, Austen KF, Soberman RJ. Leukotrienes and other products of the 5-lipoxygenase pathway. Biochemistry and relation to pathobiology in human diseases. *N Engl J Med,* 323:645–55, 1990 Sep 6.

Lipkin M, Newmark H. Calcium and the prevention of colon cancer. *J Cell Biochem,* Suppl 22:65–73, 1995.

Lipworth L, Martínez ME, Angell J, Hsieh CC, Trichopoulos D. Olive oil and human cancer: an assessment of the evidence. *Prev Med,* 26:181–90, 1997 Mar–Apr.

Malmsten CL. Arachidonic acid metabolism and inflammation. A brief introduction. *Scand J Rheumatol,* Suppl, 53:31–45, 1984.

Malmsten CL. Arachidonic acid metabolism in inflammation and hypersensitivity reactions: a brief introduction. *Cephalalgia,* 6 Suppl 4:13–16, 1986.

Malmsten CL. Prostaglandins, thromboxanes, and leukotrienes in inflammation. *Am J Med,* 80:11–17, 1986 Apr 28.

Malmsten CL. Leukotrienes: mediators of inflammation and immediate hypersensitivity reactions. *Crit Rev Immunol,* 4:307–34, 1984.

Manson JE, Stampfer MJ, Hennekens CH, Willett WC. Body weight and longevity. A reassessment. *JAMA,* 257:353–8, 1987 Jan 16.

Manson JE, Willett WC, Stampfer MJ, et al. Body weight and mortality among women [see comments]. *N Engl J Med,* 333:677–85, 1995 Sept 14.

Manson JE, Colditz GA, Stampfer MJ, et al. A prospective study of obesity and risk of coronary heart disease in women [see comments]. *N Engl J Med,* 322:882–9, 1990 Mar 29.

Margaritis I, Tessier F, Prou E, Marconnet P, Marini JF. Effects of endurance training on skeletal muscle oxidative capacities with and without selenium supplementation. *J Trace Elem Med Biol,* 11:37–43, 1997 Apr.

Marin P, Jansson S, Krotkiewski M, Holm G, Björntorp P. Uptake of glucose carbon in muscle glycogen and adipose tissue triglycerides in vivo in humans. *Am J Physiol,* 263:E473–80, 1992 Sep.

Marnett LJ, Wilcox CL. Stimulation of prostaglandin biosynthesis by lipoic acid. *Biochim Biophys Acta,* 487:222–30, 1977 Apr 26.

Marquart LF, Sobal J. Weight loss beliefs, practices and support systems for high school wrestlers. *J Adolesc Health,* 15:410–15, 1994 Jul.

Martin-Du Pan RC, Wurtman RJ. [The role of nutrition in the synthesis of neurotransmitters and in cerebral functions: clinical implications.] *Schweiz Med Wochenschr,* 111:1422–34, 1981 Sep 26.

Martin-Moreno JM, Willett WC, Gorgojo L, et al. Dietary fat, olive oil intake and breast cancer risk. *Int J Cancer,* 58:774–80, 1994 Sep 15.

Martinuzzi A, Vergani L, Rosa M, Angelini C. L-carnitine uptake in differentiating human cultured muscle. *Biochem Biophys Acta,* 1095:217–22, 1991 Nov 12.

Mataix J. Recent findings in olive oil research. *Eur J Clin Nutr,* 47 Suppl 1:S82–4, 1993 Sep.

Matkovic V, Ilich JZ, Skugor M, et al. Leptin is inversely related to age at menarche in human females. *J Clin Endocrinol Metab,* 82:3239–45, 1997 Oct.

Mattes RD. Fat preference and adherence to a reduced-fat diet. *Am J Clin Nutr,* 57:373–81, 1993 Mar.

McCarty MF. Anabolic effects of insulin on bone suggest a role for chromium picolinate in preservation of bone density. *Med Hypotheses,* 45:241–6, 1995 Sep.

McLellan TM, Jacobs I. Muscle glycogen utilization and the expression of relative exercise intensity. *Int J Sports Med,* 12:21–6, 1991 Feb.

Mee JF, Reitsma P, Mehra R. Effect of a whey protein concentrate used as a colostrum substitute or supplement on calf immunity, weight gain, and health. *J Dairy Sci,* 79:886–94, 1996 May.

Meezan E, Meezan J, Manzella S, Rodén L. Alkylglycosides as artificial primers for glycogen biosynthesis. *Cell Mol Biol* (Noisy-le-grand), 43:369–81, 1997 May.

Mela DJ. Understanding fat preference and consumption: applications of behavioural sciences to a nutritional problem. *Proc Nutr Soc,* 54:453–64, 1995 Jul.

Mela DJ, Sacchetti DA. Sensory preferences for fats: relationships with diet and body composition. *Am J Clin Nutr,* 53:908–15, 1991 Apr.

Mengeaud V, Nano JL, Fournel S, Rampal P. Effects of eicosapentaenoic acid, gamma-linolenic acid and prostaglandin E1 on three human colon carcinoma cell lines. *Prostaglandins Leukot Essent Fatty Acids,* 47:313–19, 1992.

Mensink RP, Katan MB. An epidemiological and an experimental study on the effect of olive oil on total serum and HDL cholesterol in healthy volunteers. *Eur J Clin Nutr,* 43 Suppl 2:43–8, 1989.

Mensink RP, de Groot MJ, van den Broeke LT, Severijnen-Nobels AP, Demacker PN, Katan MB. Effects of monounsaturated fatty acids v complex carbohydrates on serum lipoproteins and apoproteins in healthy men and women. *Metabolism,* 38:172–8, 1989 Feb.

Messina MJ, Persky V, Setchell KD, Barnes S. Soy intake and cancer risk: a review of the in vitro and in vivo data. *Nutr Cancer,* 21:113–31, 1994.

Metz JA, Anderson JJ, Gallagher PN, Jr. Intakes of calcium, phosphorus, and protein, and physical-activity level are related to radial bone mass in young adult women [see comments]. *Am J Clin Nutr,* 58:537–42, 1993 Oct.

Miller CC, McCreedy CA, Jones AD, Ziboh VA. Oxidative metabolism of dihomogammalinolenic acid by guinea pig epidermis: evidence of generation of anti-inflammatory products. *Prostaglandins,* 35:917–38, 1988 Jun.

Mitchell SL, Epstein LH. Changes in taste and satiety in dietary-restrained women following stress. *Physiol Behav,* 60:495–9, 1996 Aug.

Mizushima S, Moriguchi EH, Ishikawa P, et al. Fish intake and cardiovascular risk among middle-aged Japanese in Japan and Brazil. *J Cardiovasc Risk,* 4:191–9, 1997 Jun.

Mohs RC, Davis KL, Tinklenberg JR, Hollister LE, Yesavage JA, Kopell BS. Choline chloride treatment of memory deficits in the elderly. *Am J Psychiatry,* 136:1275–7, 1979 Oct.

Moore TL, Weiss TD. Mediators of inflammation. *Semin Arthritis Rheum,* 14:247–62, 1985 May.

Mullan LM, Holton EE, Vickers ZM. Preference for and consumption of fat-free and full-fat cheese by children. *J Am Diet Assoc,* 96:603–4, 1996 Jun.

Muller C, Assimacopoulos-Jeannet F, Mosimann F, et al. Endogenous glucose production, gluconeogenesis and liver glycogen concentration in obese non-diabetic patients. *Diabetologia,* 40:463–8, 1997 Apr.

Mundy GR. Cytokines and growth factors in the regulation of bone remodeling. *J Bone Miner Res,* 8 Suppl 2:S505–10, 1993 Dec.

Nagamatsu M, Nickander KK, Schmelzer JD, et al. Lipoic acid improves nerve blood flow, reduces oxidative stress, and improves distal nerve conduction in experimental diabetic neuropathy. *Diabetes Care,* 18:1160–7, 1995 Aug.

Nakatani A, Han DH, Hansen PA, et al. Effect of endurance exercise training on muscle glycogen supercompensation in rats. *J Appl Physiol,* 82:711–15, 1997 Feb.

Nakielny S, Campbell DG, Cohen P. The molecular mechanism by which adrenalin inhibits glycogen synthesis. *Eur J Biochem,* 199:713–22, 1991 Aug 1.

Nal, ecz KA, Nal, ecz MJ. Carnitine—a known compound, a novel function in neural cells. *Acta Neurobiol Exp* (Warsz), 56:597–609, 1996.

Narisawa T, Takahashi M, Kotanagi H, Kusaka H, Yamazaki Y, Koyama H. Inhibitory effect of dietary perilla oil rich in the n-3 polyunsaturated fatty acid alpha-linolenic acid on colon carcinogenesis in rats. *Jpn J Cancer Res,* 82:1089–96, 1991.

Narisawa T, Fukaura Y, Yazawa K, Ishikawa C, Isoda Y, Nishizawa Y. Colon cancer prevention with a small amount of dietary perilla oil high in alpha-linolenic acid in an animal model. *Cancer,* 73:2069–75, 1994.

Nelson RG, Sievers ML, Knowler WC, et al. Low incidence of fatal coronary heart disease in Pima Indians despite high prevalence of non-insulin-dependent diabetes. *Circulation,* 81:987–95, 1990.

Neoptolemos JP, Husband D, Imray C, Rowley S, Lawson N. Arachidonic acid and docosahexaenoic acid are increased in human colorectal cancer. *Gut,* 32:278–81, 1991.

Nettleton JA. Are n-3 fatty acids essential nutrients for fetal and infant development? *J Am Diet Assoc,* 93:58–64, 1993 Jan.

Nettleton JA. Omega-3 fatty acids: comparison of plant and seafood sources in human nutrition. *J Am Diet Assoc,* 91:331–7, 1991 Mar.

Newmark HL, Lipkin M. Calcium, vitamin D, and colon cancer. *Cancer Res,* 52:S2067–70, 1992.

Ne¨ichev K, Slavcheva E, Abrashev I, Todorova P, Mitov I, Veselinova D. [The immunomodulating properties of a glucomacropeptide from whey. I. The stimulation of resistance in mice.] *Acta Microbiol Bulg,* 25:54–61, 1990.

Nicklas BJ, Rogus EM, Goldberg AP. Exercise blunts declines in lipolysis and fat oxidation after dietary-induced weight loss in obese older women. *Am J Physiol,* 273:E149–55, 1997 Jul.

Nissen S, Fuller JC, Jr., Sell J, Ferket PR, Rives DV. The effect of beta-hydroxy-beta-methylbutyrate on growth, mortality, and carcass qualities of broiler chickens. *Poult Sci,* 73:137–55, 1994 Jan.

Nissen S, Sharp R, Ray M, et al. Effect of leucine metabolite beta-hydroxy-beta-methylbutyrate on muscle metabolism during resistance-exercise training. *J Appl Physiol,* 81:2095–104, 1996 Nov.

Nordheim K. Glycogen and lactate metabolism during low-intensity exercise in man. *Acta Physiol Scand,* 139:475–84, 1990 Jul.

O'Brien T, Nguyen TT, Buithieu J, Kottke BA. Lipoprotein compositional changes in the fasting and postprandial state on a high-carbohydrate low-fat and a high-fat diet in subjects with noninsulin-dependent diabetes mellitus. *J Clin Endocrinol Metab,* 77:1345–51, 1993 Nov.

O'Dea K, Spargo RM. Metabolic adaptation to a low carbohydrate-high protein ("traditional") diet in Australian Aborigines. *Diabetologia,* 23:494–8, 1982 Dec.

O'Dea K, Sinclair AJ. The effects of low-fat diets rich in arachidonic acid on the composition of plasma fatty acids and bleeding time in Australian aborigines. *J Nutr Sci Vitaminol* (Tokyo), 31:441–53, 1985 Aug.

Odland LM, Heigenhauser GJ, Wong D, Hollidge-Horvat MG, Spriet LL. Effects of increased fat availability on fat-carbohydrate interaction during prolonged exercise in men. *Am J Physiol,* 274:R894–902, 1998 Apr.

O'Hara W, Allen C, Shephard RJ. Loss of body fat during an arctic winter expedition. *Can J Physiol Pharmacol,* 55:1235–41, 1977 Dec.

O'Hara W, Allen C, Shephard RJ. Treatment of obesity by exercise in the cold. *Can Med Assoc J,* 117:773–8, 786, 1977 Oct 8.

Packard PT, Recker RR. Caffeine does not affect the rate of gain in spine bone in young women. *Osteoporos Int,* 6:149–52, 1996.

Pagliacci MC, Smacchia M, Migliorati G, Grignani F, Riccardi C, Nicoletti. Growth-inhibitory effects of the natural phyto-oestrogen genistein in MCF-7 human breast cancer cells. *Eur J Cancer* 30A, 11:1675–82, 1994.

Pagnan A, Corrocher R, Ambrosio GB, et al. Effects of an olive-oil-rich diet on erythrocyte membrane lipid composition and cation transport systems. *Clin Sci,* 76:87–93, 1989 Jan.

Pandalai PK, Pilat MJ, Yamazaki K, Naik H, Pienta KJ. The effects of omega-3 and omega-6 fatty acids on in vitro prostate cancer growth. *Anticancer Res,* 16:815–20, 1996.

Papet I, Ostaszewski P, Glomot F, et al. The effect of a high dose of 3-hydroxy-3-methylbutyrate on protein metabolism in growing lambs. *Br J Nutr,* 77:885–96, 1997 Jun.

Pasman WJ, van Baak MA, Jeukendrup AE, de Haan A. The effect of different dosages of caffeine on endurance performance time. *Int J Sports Med,* 16:225–30, 1995 May.

Peak M, al-Habori M, Agius L. Regulation of glycogen synthesis and glycolysis by insulin, pH and cell volume. Interactions between swelling and alkalinization in mediating the effects of insulin. *Biochem J,* 282 (Pt 3):797–805, 1992 Mar 15.

Perez C, Lucas F, Sclafani A. Carbohydrate, fat, and protein condition similar flavor preferences in rats using an oral-delay procedure. *Physiol Behav,* 57:549–54, 1995 Mar.

Perez-Jimenez F, Espino A, Lopez-Segura F, et al. Lipoprotein concentrations in normolipidemic males consuming oleic acid-rich diets from two different souces: olive oil and oleic acid-rich sunflower oil. *Am J Clin Nutr,* 62:769–75, 1995 Oct.

Peters Futre EM, Noakes TD, Raine RI, Terblanche SE. Muscle glycogen repletion during active postexercise recovery. *Am J Physiol,* 253:E305–11, 1987 Sept.

Peterson G, Barnes S. Genistein inhibits both estrogen and growth factor-stimulated proliferation of human breast cancer cells. *Cell Growth Differ,* 7:1345–51, 1996.

Petrakis NL, Barnes S, King EB, et al. Stimulatory influence of soy protein isolate on breast secretion in pre- and postmenopausal women. *Cancer Epidemiol Biomarkers Prev,* 5:785–94, 1996.

Petroni A, Blasevich M, Salami M, Papini N, Montedoro GF, Galli C. Inhibition of platelet aggregation and eicosanoid production by phenolic components of olive oil. *Thromb Res,* 78:151–60, 1995 Apr 15.

Petroni A, Blasevich M, Salami M, Servili M, Montedoro GF, Galli C. A phenolic antioxidant extracted from olive oil inhibits platelet aggregation and arachidonic acid metabolism in vitro. *World Rev Nutr Diet,* 75:169–72, 1994.

Phinney SD, Bistrian BR, Wolfe RR, Blackburn GL. The human metabolic response to chronic ketosis without caloric restriction: physical and biochemical adaptation. *Metabolism,* 32:757–68, 1983 Aug.

Piatti PM, Monti F, Fermo I, et al. Hypocaloric high-protein diet improves glucose oxidation and spares lean body mass: comparison to hypocaloric high-carbohydrate diet. *Metabolism,* 43:1481–7, 1994 Dec.

Potter SM. Soy protein and serum lipids. *Curr Opin Lipidol,* 7:260–4, 1996.

Powers SK, Criswell D. Adaptive strategies of respiratory muscles in response to endurance exercise. *Med Sci Sports Exerc,* 28:1115–22, 1996 Sep.

Preisinger E, Leitner G, Uher E, et al. [Nutrition and osteoporosis: a nutritional analysis of women in postmenopause.] *Wien Klin Wochenschr,* 107:418–22, 1995.

Prior JC, Barr SI, Chow R, Faulkner RA. Prevention and management of osteoporosis: consensus statements from the Scientific Advisory Board of the Osteoporosis Society of Canada. 5. Physical activity as therapy for osteoporosis. *CMAJ,* 155:940–4, 1996 Oct 1.

Pritchard RS, Baron JA, Gerhardsson de Verdier M. Dietary calcium, vitamin D, and the risk of colorectal cancer in Stockholm, Sweden. *Cancer Epidemiol Biomarkers Prev,* 5:897–900, 1996.

Purasiri P, Murray A, Richardson S, Heys SD, Horrobin D, Eremin O. Modulation of cytokine production in vivo by dietary essential fatty acids in patients with colorectal cancer. *Clin Sci,* 87:711–17, 1994.

Raben A, Kiens B, Richter EA, et al. Serum sex hormones and endurance performance after a lacto-ovo vegetarian and a mixed diet. *Med Sci Sports Exerc,* 24:1290–7, 1992 Nov.

Raines EW, Ross R. Biology of atherosclerotic plaque formation: possible role of growth factors in lesion development and the potential impact of soy. *J Nutr,* 125:S624–630, 1995.

Rains TM, Shay NF. Zinc status specifically changes preferences for carbohydrate and protein in rats selecting from separate carbohydrate-, protein-, and fat-containing diets. *J Nutr,* 125:2874–9, 1995 Nov.

Rao GN. Influence of diet on tumors of hormonal tissues. *Prog Clin Biol Res,* 394:41–56, 1996.

Rasmussen O, Lauszus FF, Christiansen C, Thomsen C, Hermansen K. Differential effects of saturated and monounsaturated fat on blood glucose and insulin responses in subjects with non-insulin-dependent diabetes mellitus. *Am J Clin Nutr,* 63:249–53, 1996 Feb.

Rasmussen OW, Thomsen C, Hansen KW, Vesterlund M, Winther E, Hermansen K. Effects on blood pressure, glucose, and lipid levels of a high-monounsaturated fat diet compared with a high-carbohydrate diet in NIDDM subjects. *Diabetes Care,* 16:1565–71, 1993 Dec.

Ready AE, Naimark B, Ducas J, et al. Influence of walking volume on health benefits in women post-menopause. *Med Sci Sports Exerc,* 28:1097–105, 1996 Sep.

Reichmann H, van Lindeneiner N. Carnitine analysis in normal human red blood cells, plasma, and muscle tissue. *Eur Neurol,* 34:40–3, 1994.

Reinli K, Block G. Phytoestrogen content of foods—a compendium of literature values. *Nutr Cancer,* 26:123–48, 1996.

Ren JM, Broberg S, Sahlin K, Hultman E. Influence of reduced glycogen level on glycogenolysis during short-term stimulation in man. *Acta Physiol Scand,* 139:467–74, 1990 Jul.

Ricketts CD. Fat preferences, dietary fat intake and body composition in children. *Eur J Clin Nutr,* 51:778–81, 1997 Nov.

Robertson TL, Kato H, Rhoads GG, et al. Epidemiologic studies of coronary heart disease and stroke in Japanese men living in Japan, Hawaii and California. Incidence of myocardial infarction and death from coronary heart disease. *Am J Cardiol,* 39:239–43, 1977 Feb.

Roche HM, Zampelas A, Knapper JM, et al. Effect of long-term olive oil dietary intervention on postprandial triacylglycerol and factor VII metabolism. *Am J Clin Nutr,* 68:552–60, 1998 Sep.

Rockwood GA, Bhathena SJ. High-fat diet preference in developing and adult rats. *Physiol Behav,* 48:79–82, 1990 Jul.

Rohan TE, Howe GR, Burch JD, Jain M. Dietary factors and risk of prostate cancer: a case-control study in Ontario, Canada. *Cancer Causes Control,* 6:145–54, 1995.

Rolls BJ, Miller DL. Is the low-fat message giving people a license to eat more? *J Am Coll Nutr,* 16:535–43, 1997 Dec.

Rose DP, Cohen LA. Effects of dietary menhaden oil and retinyl acetate on the growth of DU 145 human prostatic adenocarcinoma cells transplanted into athymic nude mice. *Carcinogenesis,* 9:603–5, 1988.

Rosen JC, Gross J, Loew D, Sims EA. Mood and appetite during minimal-carbohydrate and carbohydrate-supplemented hypocaloric diets. *Am J Clin Nutr,* 42:371–9, 1985 Sep.

Rosen CJ, Donahue LR, Hunter SJ. Insulin-like growth factors and bone: the osteoporosis connection. *Proc Soc Exp Biol Med,* 206:83–102, 1994 Jun.

Ross R, L Le, Marliss EB, Morris DV, Gougeon R. Adipose tissue distribution changes during rapid weight loss in obese adults. *Int J Obes,* 15:733–9, 1991 Nov.

Roth E. Oxygen free radicals and their clinical implications. *Acta Chir Hung,* 36:302–5, 1997.

Roust LR, Kottke BA, Jensen MD. Serum lipid responses to a eucaloric high-complex carbohydrate diet in different obesity phenotypes. *Mayo Clin Proc,* 69:930–6, 1994 Oct.

Rudolf MC, Sherwin RS. Maternal ketosis and its effects on the fetus. *Clin Endocrinol Metab,* 12:413–28, 1983 Jul.

Ruiz-Gutíerrez V, Morgado N, Prada JL, Pe-Je F, Muriana FJ. Composition of human VLDL triacylglycerols after ingestion of olive oil and high oleic sunflower oil. *J Nutr,* 128:570–6, 1998 Mar.

Ryan AS, Pratley RE, Goldberg AP, Elahi D. Resistive training increases insulin action in postmenopausal women. *J Gerontol A Biol Sci Med Sci,* 51:M199–205, 1996 Sept.

Ryan AS, Pratley RE, Elahi D, Goldberg AP. Resistive training increases fat-free mass and maintains RMR despite weight loss in postmenopausal women. *J Appl Physiol,* 79:818–23, 1995 Sep.

Saad MF, Lillioja S, Nyomba BL, Castillo C, Ferraro R, De Gregorio M. Racial differences in the relation between blood pressure and insulin resistance. *N Engl J Med,* 324:733–9, 1991.

Safer DJ. Diet, behavior modification, and exercise: a review of obesity treatments from a long-term perspective. *South Med J,* 84:1470–4, 1991 Dec.

Sahlin K. Muscle carnitine metabolism during incremental dynamic exercise in humans. *Acta Physiol Scand,* 138:259–62, 1990 Mar.

Saitoh S, Matsuo T, Tagami K, Chang H, Tokuyama K, Suzuki M. Effects of short-term dietary change from high fat to high carbohydrate diets on the storage and utilization of glycogen and triacylglycerol in untrained rats. *Eur J Appl Physiol,* 74:13–22, 1996.

Salyers AA, Sperry JF, Wilkins TD, Walker AR, Richardson NJ. Neutral steroid concentrations in the faeces of North American White and South African Black populations at different risks for cancer of the colon. *SB:M. S Afr Med J,* 51:823–7, 1977.

Samuelsson B. Arachidonic acid metabolism: role in inflammation. *Z Rheumatol,* 50 Suppl 1:3–6, 1991.

Samuelsson B. An elucidation of the arachidonic acid cascade. Discovery of prostaglandins, thromboxane and leukotrienes. *Drugs,* 33 Suppl 1:2–9, 1987.

Samuelsson B. Leukotrienes: a new class of mediators of immediate hypersensitivity reactions and inflammation. *Adv Prostaglandin Thromboxane Leukot Res,* 11:1–13, 1983.

Sanchez CJ, Hooper E, Garry PJ, Goodwin JM, Goodwin JS. The relationship between dietary intake of choline, choline serum levels, and cognitive function in healthy elderly persons. *J Am Geriatr Soc,* 32:208–12, 1984 Mar.

Satabin P, Bois-Joyeux B, Chanez M, Guezennec CY, Peret J. Post-exercise glycogen resynthesis in trained high-protein or high-fat-fed rats after glucose feeding. *Eur J Appl Physiol,* 58:591–5, 1989.

Schaefer EJ, Lichtenstein AH, Lamon-Fava S, et al. Body weight and low-density lipoprotein cholesterol changes after consumption of a low-fat ad libitum diet [see comments]. *JAMA,* 274:1450–5, 1995 Nov 8.

Schürch MA, Rizzoli R, Slosman D, Vadas L, Vergnaud P, Bonjour JP. Protein supplements increase serum insulin-like growth factor-I levels and attenuate proximal femur bone loss in patients with recent hip fracture. A randomized, double-blind, placebo-controlled trial. *Ann Intern Med,* 128:801–9, 1998 May 15.

Schutz Y, Flatt JP. Failure of dietary fat intake to promote fat oxidation: a factor favoring the development of obesity [see comments]. *Am J Clin Nutr,* 50:307–14, 1989 Aug.

Sclafani A, Ackroff K. Deprivation alters rats' flavor preferences for carbohydrates and fats. *Physiol Behav,* 53:1091–9, 1993 Jun.

Serra F, Diaspri GP, Gasbarrini A, et al. [Effect of CDP-choline on senile mental deterioration. Multicenter experience on 237 cases.] *Minerva Med,* 81:465–70, 1990 Jun.

Shi X, Gisolfi, CV. Fluid and carbohydrate replacement during intermittent exercise. *Sports Med,* 25:157–72, 1998.

Sinclair AJ, Johnson L, Holman RT. Diets rich in lean beef increase arachidonic acid and long-chain omega 3 polyunsaturated fatty acid levels in plasma phospholipids. *Lipids,* 29:337–43, 1994 May.

Siow BL. Cerebral ageing, neurotransmitters and therapeutic implications. *Singapore Med J,* 26:151–3, 1985 Apr.

Sirtori CR, Tremoli E, Gatti E, et al. Controlled evaluation of fat intake in the Mediterranean diet: comparative activities of olive oil and corn oil on plasma lipids and platelets in high-risk patients. *Am J Clin Nutr,* 44:635–42, 1986 Nov.

Sirtori CR, Gatti E, Tremoli E, et al. Olive oil, corn oil, and n-3 fatty acids differently affect lipids, lipoproteins, platelets, and superoxide formation in type II hypercholesterolemia. *Am J Clin Nutr,* 56:113–22, 1992 Jul.

Sitaram N, Weingartner H, Caine ED, Gillin JC. Choline: Selective enhancement of serial learning and encoding of low imagery words in man. *Life Sci,* 22:1555–60, 1978 May 1.

Sitton SC. Role of craving for carbohydrates upon completion of a protein-sparing fast. *Psychol Rep,* 69:683–6, 1991 Oct.

Skutches CL, Owen OE, Reichard GA, Jr. Acetone and acetol inhibition of insulin-stimulated glucose oxidation in adipose tissue and isolated adipocytes. *Diabetes,* 39:450–5, 1990 Apr.

Smith U. Carbohydrates, fat, and insulin action. *Am J Clin Nutr,* 59:S686–9, 1994 Mar.

So FV, Guthrie N, Chambers AF, Moussa M, Carroll KK. Inhibition of human breast cancer cell proliferation and delay of mammary tumorigenesis by flavonoids and citrus juices. *Nutr Cancer,* 26:167–81, 1996.

Solomon CG, Manson JE. Obesity and mortality: a review of the epidemiologic data. *Am J Clin Nutr,* 66:S1044–50, 1997 Oct.

Sossin K, Gizis F, Marquart LF, Sobal J. Nutrition beliefs, attitudes, and resource use of high school wrestling coaches. *Int J Sport Nutr,* 7:219–28, 1997 Sept.

Souba WWRJS, Wilmore DW. Glutamine metabolism by the intestinal tract. *JPEN J. Parenter. Enteral. Nutr.,* 9:608–17, 1985.

Spagnoli LG, Palmieri G, Mauriello A, et al. Morphometric evidence of the trophic effect of L-carnitine on human skeletal muscle. *Nephron,* 55:16–23, 1990.

Sparti A. Effect of diet on glucose tolerance 36 hours after glycogen-depleting exercise. *Eur J Clin Nutr,* 46:377–85, 1992 Jun.

Spina RJ, Ogawa T, Kohrt WM, Martin WH 3d, Holloszy JO, Ehsani AA. Differences in cardiovascular adaptations to endurance exercise training between older men and women. *J Appl Physiol,* 75:849–55, 1993 Aug.

Spriet LL, Peters SJ. Influence of diet on the metabolic responses to exercise. *Proc Nutr Soc,* 57:25–33, 1998 Feb.

Stacpoole PW. Should NIDDM patients be on high-carbohydrate, low-fat diets? Affirmative [see comments]. *Hosp Pract (Off Ed),* 27 Suppl 1:6–10; discussion 14-6, 1992 Feb.

Stallings VA, Pencharz PB. The effect of a high protein–low calorie diet on the energy expenditure of obese adolescents. *Eur J Clin Nutr,* 46:897–902, 1992 Dec.

Stanko RT, Tietze DL, Arch JE. Body composition, energy utilization, and nitrogen metabolism with a severely restricted diet supplemented with dihydroxyacetone and pyruvate. *Am J Clin Nutr,* 55:771–6, 1992 Apr.

Stanko RT, Tietze DL, Arch JE. Body composition, energy utilization, and nitrogen metabolism with a 4.25-MJ/d low-energy diet supplemented with pyruvate. *Am J Clin Nutr,* 56:630–5, 1992 Oct.

Stanko RT et al. Plasma lipid concentrations in hyperlipidemic patients consuming a high-fat diet supplemented with pyruvate for six weeks. *Am J Clin Nutr,* 56:950–4, 1992.

Stanko RT et al. Pyruvate supplementation of a low-cholesterol, low-fat diet: effects on plasma lipid concentrations and body composition in hyperlipidemic patients. *Am J Clin Nutr,* 59:423–7, 1994.

Starling RD, Costill DL, Fink WJ. Relationships between muscle carnitine, age and oxidative status. *Eur J Appl Physiol,* 71:143–6, 1995.

Stemmermann GN. Patterns of disease among Japanese living in Hawaii. *Arch Environ Health,* 20:266–73, 1970 Feb.

Stern MP, Haffner SM. Body fat distribution and hyperinsulinemia as risk factors for diabetes and cardiovascular disease. *Arteriosclerosis,* 6:123–30, 1986.

Stevenson RW, Mitchell DR, Hendrick GK, Rainey R, Cherrington AD, Frizzell RT. Lactate as substrate for glycogen resynthesis after exercise. *J Appl Physiol,* 62:2237–40, 1987 Jun.

Suzuki YJ, Tsuchiya M, Packer L. Lipoate prevents glucose-induced protein modifications. *Free Radic Res Commun,* 17:211–17, 1992.

Takada Y, Kobayashi N, Kato K, Matsuyama H, Yahiro M, Aoe S. Effects of whey protein on calcium and bone metabolism in ovariectomized rats. *J Nutr Sci Vitaminol* (Tokyo), 43:199–210, 1997 Apr.

Talmadge RJ, Silverman H. Glyconeogenic and glycogenic enzymes in chronically active and normal skeletal muscle. *J Appl Physiol,* 71:182–91, 1991 Jul.

Tanaka H, Swensen T. Impact of resistance training on endurance performance. A new form of cross-training? *Sports Med,* 25:191–200, 1998 Mar.

Tataranni PA, Larson DE, Snitker S, Young JB, Flatt JP, Ravussin E. Effects of glucocorticoids on energy metabolism and food intake in humans. *Am J Physiol,* 271:E317–25, 1996 Aug.

Tepper BJ, Friedman MI. Altered acceptability of and preference for sugar solutions by diabetic rats is normalized by high-fat diet. *Appetite,* 16:25–38, 1991 Feb.

Tew BY, Xu X, Wang HJ, Murphy PA, Hendrich S. A diet high in wheat fiber decreases the bioavailability of soybean isoflavones in a single meal fed to women. *J Nutr,* 126:871–7, 1996.

Tiggemann M. Dietary restraint as a predictor of reported weight loss and affect. *Psychol Rep,* 75:1679–82, 1994 Dec.

Tisdale MJ. Inhibition of lipolysis and muscle protein degradation by EPA in cancer cachexia. *Nutrition,* 12:S31–3, 1996.

Toornvliet AC, Pijl H, Frölich M, Westendorp RG, Meinders AE. Insulin and leptin concentrations in obese humans during long-term weight loss. *Neth J Med,* 51:96–102, 1997 Sept.

Trichopoulou A, Katsouyanni K, Stuver S, et al. Consumption of olive oil and specific food groups in relation to breast cancer risk in Greece [see comments]. *J Natl Cancer Inst,* 87:110–16, 1995 Jan 18.

Truswell AS, Choudhury N. Monounsaturated oils do not all have the same effect on plasma cholesterol. *Eur J Clin Nutr,* 52:312–15, 1998 May.

Truswell AS. Food carbohydrates and plasma lipids—an update. *Am J Clin Nutr,* 59:S710–18, 1994 Mar.

Tuominen JA, Peltonen JE, Koivisto VA. Blood flow, lipid oxidation, and muscle glycogen synthesis after glycogen depletion by strenuous exercise. *Med Sci Sports Exerc,* 29:874–81, 1997 Jul.

Tuominen JA, Ebeling P, Vuorinen-Markkola H, Koivisto VA. Post-marathon paradox in IDDM: unchanged insulin sensitivity in spite of glycogen depletion. *Diabet Med,* 14:301–8, 1997 Apr.

Tyler DO, Allan JD, Alcozer FR. Weight loss methods used by African American and Euro-American women. *Res Nurs Health,* 20:413–23, 1997 Oct.

Tzonou A, Hsieh CC, Polychronopoulou A, Kaprinis G, Toupadaki N. Diet and ovarian cancer: a case-control study in Greece. *Int J Cancer,* 55:411–114, 1993.

Ullmann D, Connor WE, Hatcher LF, Connor SL, Flavell DP. Will a high-carbohydrate, low-fat diet lower plasma lipids and lipoproteins without producing hypertriglyceridemia? *Arterioscler Thromb,* 11:1059–67, 1991 Jul–Aug.

Urhausen A, Kindermann W. Blood ammonia and lactate concentrations during endurance exercise of differing intensities. *Eur J Appl Physiol,* 65:209–14, 1992.

Van Aswegen CH, Du Plessis DJ. Can linoleic acid and gamma-linolenic acid be important in cancer treatment? *Med Hypotheses,* 43:415–17, 1994.

Van de Stadt KD. Prostaglandins and leukotrienes in inflammation and allergy. *Neth J Med,* 25:22–9, 1982.

van der Merwe CF, Booyens J, Joubert HF, van der Merwe CA. The effect of gamma-linolenic acid, an in vitro cytostatic substance contained in evening primrose oil, on primary liver cancer. A double-blind placebo controlled trial. *Prostaglandins Leukot Essent Fatty Acids,* 40:199–202, 1990.

Varnier M, Leese GP, Thompson J, Rennie MJ. Stimulatory effect of glutamine on glycogen accumulation in human skeletal muscle. *Am J Physiol,* 269:E309–15, 1995 Aug.

Vazquez JA, Kazi U, Madani N. Protein metabolism during weight reduction with very-low-energy diets: evaluation of the independent effects of protein and carbohydrate on protein sparing. *Am J Clin Nutr,* 62:93–103, 1995 Jul.

Vergauwen L, Richter EA, Hespel P. Adenosine exerts a glycogen-sparing action in contracting rat skeletal muscle. *Am J Physiol,* 272:E762–8, 1997 May.

Vicario IM, Malkova D, Lund EK, Johnson IT. Olive oil supplementation in healthy adults: effects in cell membrane fatty acid composition and platelet function. *Ann Nutr Metab,* 42:160–9, 1998.

Villar-Palasí C, Guinovart JJ. The role of glucose 6-phosphate in the control of glycogen synthase. *FASEB J,* 11:544–58, 1997 Jun.

Visioli F, Bellomo G, Galli C. Free radical-scavenging properties of olive oil polyphenols. *Biochem Biophys Res Commun,* 247:60–4, 1998 Jun 9.

Visioli F, Bellomo G, Montedoro G, Galli C. Low density lipoprotein oxidation is inhibited in vitro by olive oil constituents. *Atherosclerosis,* 117:25–32, 1995 Sep.

Vognild E, Elvevoll EO, Brox J, et al. Effects of dietary marine oils and olive oil on fatty acid composition, platelet membrane fluidity, platelet responses, and serum lipids in healthy humans. *Lipids,* 33:427–36, 1998 Apr.

Vukovich MD, Sharp RL, Kesl LD, Schaulis DL, King DS. Effects of a low-dose amino acid supplement on adaptations to cycling training in untrained individuals. *Int J Sport Nutr,* 7:298–309, 1997 Dec.

Wadden TA, Considine RV, Foster GD, Anderson DA, Sarwer DB, Caro JS. Short- and long-term changes in serum leptin dieting obese women: effects of caloric restriction and weight loss. *J Clin Endocrinol Metab,* 83:214–18, 1998 Jan.

Wainfan E, Poirier LA. Methyl groups in carcinogenesis: effects on DNA methylation and gene expression. *Cancer Res,* 52:S2071–7, 1992.

Wang TT, Sathyamoorthy N, Phang JM. Molecular effects of genistein on estrogen receptor mediated pathways. *Carcinogenesis,* 17:271–5, 1996.

Warwick ZS, Schiffman SS, Anderson JJ. Relationship of dietary fat content to food preferences in young rats. *Physiol Behav,* 48:581–6, 1990 Nov.

Weber PC. The modification of the arachidonic acid cascade by n-3 fatty acids. *Adv Prostaglandin Thromboxane Leukot Res,* 20:232–40, 1990.

Weber P. Management of osteoporosis: is there a role for vitamin K? *Int J Vitam Nutr Res,* 67:350–6, 1997.

Weintraub MS, Rosen Y, Otto R, Eisenberg S, Breslow JL. Physical exercise conditioning in the absence of weight loss reduces fasting and postprandial triglyceride-rich lipoprotein levels. *Circulation,* 79:1007–14, 1989 May.

Weissmann G. Pathways of arachidonate oxidation to prostaglandins and leukotrienes. *Semin Arthritis Rheum,* 13:123–9, 1983 Aug.

Wenzel SE. Arachidonic acid metabolites: mediators of inflammation in asthma. *Pharmacotherapy,* 17:S3–12, 1997 Jan–Feb.

West DW, Slattery ML, Robison LM, French TK, Mahoney AW. Adult dietary intake and prostate cancer risk in Utah: a case-control study with special emphasis on aggressive tumors. *Cancer Causes Control,* 2:85–94, 1991.

Williams KI, Higgs GA. Eicosanoids and inflammation. *J Pathol,* 156:101–10, 1988 Oct.

Williamson JR, Hoffmann PL, Kohrt WM, Spina RJ, Coggan AR, Holloszy O. Endurance exercise training decreases capillary basement membrane width in older nondiabetic and diabetic adults. *J Appl Physiol,* 80:747–53, 1996 Mar.

Winblad B, Hardy J, Nilsson LG. Memory function and brain biochemistry in normal aging and in senile dementia. *Ann NY Acad Sci,* 444:255–68, 1985.

Wing RR, Vazquez JA, Ryan CM. Cognitive effects of ketogenic weight-reducing diets. *Int J Obes Relat Metab Disord,* 19:811–16, 1995 Nov.

Wolz P, Krieglstein J. Neuroprotective effects of alpha-lipoic acid and its enantiomers demonstrated in rodent models of focal cerebral ischemia. *Neuropharmacology,* 35:369–75, 1996 Mar.

Wong CW, Liu AH, Regester GO, Francis GL, Watson DL. Influence of whey and purified whey proteins on neutrophil functions in sheep. *J Dairy Res,* 64:281–8, 1997 May.

Wong CW, Watson DL. Immunomodulatory effects of dietary whey proteins in mice. *J Dairy Res,* 62:359–68, 1995 May.

Wood PD, Terry RB, Haskell WL. Metabolism of substrates: diet, lipoprotein metabolism, and exercise. *Fed Proc,* 44:358–63, 1985 Feb.

Wright PD, Rich AJ. Ketosis and nitrogen excretion in undernourished surgical patients. *Acta Chir Scand Suppl,* 507:41–8, 1981.

Wroble RR, Moxley DP. Weight loss patterns and success rates in high school wrestlers. *Med Sci Sports Exerc,* 30:625–8, 1998 Apr.

Wurtman RJ. Nutrients that modify brain function. *Sci Am,* 246:50–9, 1982 Apr.

Wuster C, Blum WF, Schlemilch S, Ranke MB, Ziegler R. Decreased serum levels of insulin-like growth factors and IGF binding protein 3 in osteoporosis. *J Intern Med,* 234:249–55, 1993 Sept.

Xu X, Harris KS, Wang HJ, Murphy PA, Hendrich S. Bioavailability of soybean isoflavones depends upon gut microflora in women. *J Nutr,* 125:2307–15, 1995.

Yam D, Eliraz A, Berry EM. Diet and disease—the Israeli paradox: possible dangers of a high omega-6 polyunsaturated fatty acid diet. *Isr J Med Sci,* 32(11):1134–43, 1996.

Yan Z, Spencer MK, Katz A. Effect of low glycogen on glycogen synthase in human muscle during and after exercise. *Acta Physiol Scand,* 145:345–52, 1992 Aug.

Yanagibori R, Suzuki Y, Kawakubo K, Makita Y, Gunji A. Carbohydrate and lipid metabolism after 20 days of bed rest. *Acta Physiol Scand Suppl,* 616:51–7, 1994.

Yaqoob P, Knapper JA, Webb DH, Williams CM, Newsholme EA, Calder PC. Effect of olive oil on immune function in middle-aged men. *Am J Clin Nutr,* 67:129–35, 1998 Jan.

Yarrows SA. Weight loss through dehydration in amateur wrestling. *J Am Diet Assoc,* 88:491–3, 1988 Apr.

Yavelow J, Finlay TH, Kennedy AR, Troll W. Bowman-Birk soybean protease inhibitor as an anticarcinogen. *Cancer Res,* 43:S2454–9, 1983.

Yoshida T, Sakane N, Umekawa T, Kondo M. Relationship between basal metabolic rate, thermogenic response to caffeine, and body weight loss following combined low calorie and exercise treatment in obese women. *Int J Obes Relat Metab Disord,* 18:345–50, 1994 May.

Young SN. Behavioral effects of dietary neurotransmitter precursors: basic and clinical aspects. *Neurosci Biobehav Rev,* 20:313–23, 1996 Summer.

Young VR. Soy protein in relation to human protein and amino acid nutrition. *J Am Diet Assoc,* 91:828–35, 1991.

Zureik M, Ducimetière P, Warnet JM, Orssaud G. Fatty acid proportions in cholesterol esters and risk of premature death from cancer in middle aged French men [see comments]. *Brit Med J,* 311:1251–4, 1995.

INDEX

CONVERSION CHART

EQUIVALENT IMPERIAL AND METRIC MEASUREMENTS

American cooks use standard containers, the 8-ounce cup and a tablespoon that takes exactly 16 level fillings to fill that cup level. Measuring by cup makes it very difficult to give weight equivalents, as a cup of densely packed butter will weigh considerably more than a cup of flour. The easiest way therefore to deal with cup measurements in recipes is to take the amount by volume rather than by weight. Thus the equation reads:

1 cup = 240 ml = 8 fl. oz.
½ up = 120 ml = 4 fl. oz.

It is possible to buy a set of American cup measures in major stores around the world.

In the States, butter is often measured in sticks. One stick is the equivalent of 8 tablespoons. One tablespoon of butter is therefore the equivalent to ½ ounce/15 grams.

Liquid Measures

Fluid Ounces	U.S.	Imperial	Milliliters
	1 tsp	1 tsp	5
¼	2 tsps	1 dessertspoon	10
½	1 tb	1 tbn	14
1	2 tbs	2 tbs	28
2	¼ cup	4 tbs	56
4	½ cup		110
5		¼ pt or 1 gill	140
6	¾ cup		170
8	1 cup		225
9			250, ¼ liter
10	1¼ cups	½ pt	280
12	1½ cups		340
15		¾ pt	420
16	2 cups		450
18	2¼ cups		500, ½ liter
20	2½ cups	1 pt	560
24	3 cups or 1½ pts		675
25		1¼ pts	700
27	3½ cups		750, ¾ liter
30	3¾ cups	1½ pts	840
32	4 cups or 2 pts or 1 qt		900
35		1¾ pts	980
36	4½ cups		1000, 1 liter
40	5 cups	2 pts or 1 qt	1120

Solid Measures

U.S. and Imperial		Metric	
Ounces	Pounds	Grams	Kilos
1		28	
2		56	
3½		100	
4	¼	112	
5		140	
6		168	
8	½	225	
9		250	¼
12	¾	340	
16	1	450	

Oven Temperature Equivalents

F	C	Gas Mark	Description
225	110	¼	Cool
250	130	½	
275	140	1	Very Slow
300	150	2	
325	170	3	Slow
350	180	4	Moderate
375	190	5	
400	200	6	Moderately Hot
425	220	7	Fairly Hot
450	230	8	Hot
475	240	9	Very Hot
500	250	10	Extremely Hot

Any broiling recipes can be used with the grill of the oven, but beware of high-temperature grills.

Equivalents for Ingredients

all-purpose flour—plain flour
arugula—rocket
beet—beetroot
coarse salt—kitchen salt
cornstarch—cornflour
eggplant—aubergine
fava beans—broad beans
granulated sugar—caster sugar
lima beans—broad beans
scallion—spring onion
shortening—white fat
snow pea—mangetout
squash—courgettes or marrow
unbleached flour—strong, white flour
zest—rind
zucchini—courgettes or marrow
baking sheet—oven tray
plastic wrap—cling film